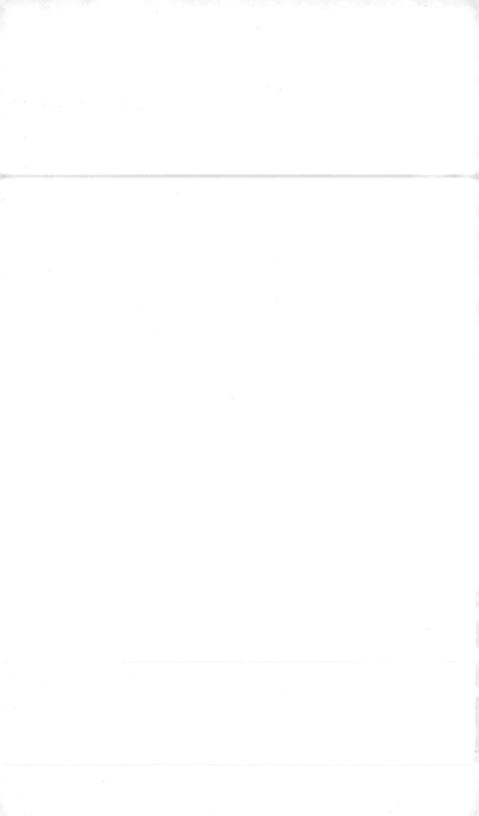

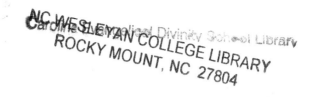
Learning to Learn

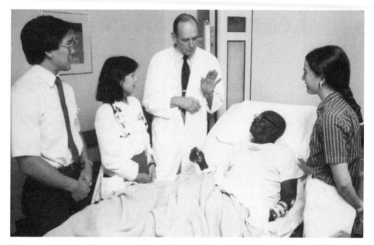

Eugene A. Stead on rounds at Duke Hospital, circa 1985, with medical students Gregory Chow, Serena Chen, and Junior Assistant Resident Kathy Merritt. Dr. Stead's copy is inscribed by Kathy Merrit: "Your challenge to learn is a true gift. Many thanks."

Learning to Learn

The Teaching Legacy of Eugene A. Stead, Jr., MD

Francis A. Neelon, MD
E. Harvey Estes, MD
Andrew G. Wallace, MD

CAROLINA ACADEMIC PRESS
Durham, North Carolina

Library of Congress Cataloging-in-Publication Data
Learning to learn : the teaching legacy of Eugene A. Stead, Jr.,
M.D. / [edited by] Francis A. Neelon, E. Harvey Estes, Andrew G.
Wallace.
    p. ; cm.
This monograph represents the editors' attempt to capture the
essence of a day-long symposium held at the Sheraton Imperial
Hotel in Research Triangle Park, North Carolina, on October 26,
2008 in honor of the 100th anniversary of the birth of Eugene A.
Stead Jr.
Includes bibliographical references and index.
ISBN 978-1-59460-841-4 (alk. paper)
    1. Medical education--Congresses. 2. Stead, Eugene A.--Con-
gresses. I. Neelon, Francis A. II. Estes, E. Harvey (Edward Har-
vey), 1925- III. Wallace, Andrew G., 1935- IV. Title.
    [DNLM: 1. Stead, Eugene A. 2. Duke University. School of
Medicine. 3. Physicians--Congresses. 4. Medicine--Congresses.
5. Schools, Medical--Congresses. 6. Teaching--methods--Con-
gresses. WZ 100 S799c 2010]

    R735.A2L43 2010
    610.71'173--dc22

                                           2010002885

CAROLINA ACADEMIC PRESS
700 Kent Street
Durham, North Carolina 27701
Telephone (919) 489-7486
Fax (919) 493-5668
www.cap-press.com

Contents

Preface

On October 26, 2008, a group of Eugene Stead's former pupils and colleagues, largely drawn from the medical and physician assistant communities, assembled for a day-long symposium in honor of the 100th anniversary of Stead's birth. The meeting was dedicated to clarifying and preserving Stead's legacy as a teacher. After an introductory essay by Andy Wallace, six subsequent speakers focused on an aspect of that legacy. Each speaker gave an oral précis of a previously written paper, which was distributed in advance to those attending the seminar. Following each paper, 50 minutes was devoted to comments from an invited panel of commentators and from the general audience. We recorded those comments, and an edited transcript follows each of the papers in this volume.

Readers will note responses from three types of attendees: 1) medical doctors who worked directly with or under Stead, 2) medical educators who were influenced obliquely by Stead's teaching style or who were at the conference representing nearby medical institutions (University of North Carolina, Wake Forest University and East Carolina University), and 3) physician assistants or nurses who spoke to Stead's influence on those professions. The transcribed comments are inserted following the nominal topic that preceded them, but readers will note instances in which speakers refer to topics that were presented earlier or were scheduled for later presentation (papers were available in advance). The result is a somewhat "choppy" series of comments that are best read with the recognition that the antecedents to which they refer may not be immediate but that all are relevant to the theme of Eugene Stead's Legacy.

Acknowledgments

We acknowledge with great gratitude financial assistance from the Carnegie Corporation of New York, the Mary Duke Biddle, the Robert Wood Johnson, and the Verner Foundations, the Duke Endowment, and the Jewish Foundation of Greensboro, whose support allowed the undertaking of the symposium and the publication of this volume.

We also thank Galen Wagner, Adonna Thompson, Bud Shelton, Erin Wilson, Jim Mau, who helped in the planning of the symposium. We are grateful to Mike Borden, Executive Director and Erin McClure, Director of Conference Services, of the North Carolina Academy of Physician Assistants for their help with fund-raising and with planning and providing logistical support for the symposium, and to Kevin Bayes, Executive Director of the Society for the Preservation of Physician Assistant History and Robert Johnston, CFO and Sr. Vice President of Finance of the American Academy of Physician Assistants for help in managing our finances. A special note of thanks to Reggie Carter and the Society for the Preservation of PA History for initiating and sustaining the effort needed to accomplish this undertaking.

Learning to Learn

Chapter 1

Passing on the Stead Legacy

Andrew G. Wallace, MD

Eugene A. Stead Jr., MD (Gene) was a teacher who made a difference. He made a difference to contemporaries who worked with him, to those who later trained under him, and to the atmosphere of scholarship he helped create, first at Emory and later at Duke University. Remembrances are understandably personal. So if you ask a large number of individuals how they remember Dr. Stead, their responses will differ. However, like several notable people who preceded him, Dr. Stead also is remembered for succinct expressions of opinion or truth or wisdom, affectionately called "Steadisms." When considered together those aphorisms describe the experience of working with Dr. Stead and they describe a pattern of thinking that was both unique to him and ahead of its time. That pattern, its profound influence on others, and its special and continuing importance to any institution dedicated to educating health professionals is his legacy. That is what he gave to us and that is what we have a responsibility to capture, articulate, reaffirm, and pass on.

The goal of this essay is to outline Dr. Stead's legacy and its basis. However, I want to begin with a short account intended to provide both an orientation to what follows and an alert to what was so special. Every word in the "Sketch" below (and in the indented paragraphs that follow) is either a direct quote from Dr. Stead or a paraphrase of one of his aphorisms, altered only to put it in the *first person*.

A Sketch

In any educational institution the *primary* product is
molded and trained [students]. A person capable of
reading books written in many different languages, a
person experienced in the manipulation of ideas, a person capable of using this background for the identification and solution of now-solvable problems; these are
the most important results of an educational system.[1] I
cannot teach you anything; I can only provide the setting in which you can learn.[2] I never lecture at Duke; I
focus on attitudes because everybody else is teaching
facts.[3] Students, interns, and residents come to us for
training, but each is different and each gains satisfaction in a different way.[4] The main thing for students to
get out of medical school is a feeling of satisfaction with
medicine.[5] By education and training we attempt to recognize within individuals those areas [of their brains] that
are structured in such a way that learning is easy and
those areas where learning will occur only with a large
input of energy.[6] Because the medical profession is made
up of many different kinds of people, our goal is to identify the best use of the man and to find the limits imposed
by his structure.[7] The appreciation that behavior has a
structural basis also is useful to the physician as he or she
approaches patients. A doctor appreciates that habits
are structurally determined and once formed they are
modified with difficulty.[8] I've always felt a teacher must
be genuinely interested in others to teach.[9]

Dr. Stead's legacy begins with the first sentence in this sketch; he regarded people as the primary product of an educational institution
and his highest priority as a teacher was to help people learn: learn
about medicine, learn about how to learn, learn about themselves,
and learn about others. His focus was on learners and learning
rather than teaching.

The Early Years[10]

This piece of prose is not a biography of Gene Stead. However, a few stories about his early life are highly relevant to my message. Gene was unusually bright! He began school at the second grade level after his eight-year-old sister convinced his teachers that she had already taught him everything he could have learned in first grade. Gene didn't particularly like school, but he learned that he could cram for two or three days and pass exams with nearly perfect scores. He used his time instead to read on his own; six or seven books in a typical week, and when he was absorbed in something that interested him nothing else mattered. He graduated from high school at age sixteen, the top student in his class of fifty. He got a scholarship to Emory University where he spent much of his time as a paid assistant in the laboratory of a highly inspiring professor. Again, he crammed for exams and got grades of 98–100. But he was aware even then that a week after exams he could remember little or nothing of what he had memorized: the fallibility of short-term memory for facts not used was clear to him and remained a life-long focus of his attention.

Gene entered Emory Medical School at age twenty: "because it was tough and his competitive spirit wanted a challenge." The last two years there consisted of clerkships at Grady Hospital, where students had more responsibility for patients than at almost any other place in the country. Gene loved it and he thrived on hard work. He lived in the hospital, saw an enormous number of patients, and even as a student he delivered more babies than the Professor of Obstetrics. He served a medical internship at the Peter Bent Brigham Hospital in Boston, followed by a fellowship, followed by an internship in surgery there, followed by two years of medical residency at Cincinnati. He then returned to Boston City Hospital for two years as an Assistant in Medicine. While most of his contemporaries entered practice either directly from medical school or after one year of internship, Gene devoted seven years to intensive clinical training and it showed. He became an expert clinician.

Gene Stead's legacy as a great teacher is rooted in his way of thinking. While that way of thinking was special, his ability to influence others was predicated on the respect he commanded because of his expertise as a clinician. Respect was evident early in his career, and had he not enjoyed that respect from contemporaries and mentors (and later from students, house staff, and colleagues), many of his sometime *maverick* ideas would have gotten him into more trouble than they did. John Hickam described Gene this way: "He had a special presence ... the most attractive [and] compelling intellectual feature of Dr. Stead has always been his tremendous ability to analyze a complicated problem, reduce it to essentials, and express it with clarity."[1] John Horton put it another way: "People respect, admire, and love Dr. Stead because within the turmoil of his life he seems to have a simplicity, directness and detachment which makes him able to be calm and helpful. ... In times when most men are so selfish, his qualities of selflessness loom large. When speaking with him, I was struck by his existential state. He seemed to be deeply concentrated within himself [yet] able to be fully in the moment."[1] Words like: presence, intellect, clarity, directness, calmness, and selflessness are not commonly used, especially together, to describe someone unless that person commands tremendous respect.

Expertise

Several years ago I read a report by *The Committee on Developments in the Science of Learning,* sponsored by the National Research Council (NRC) and titled *How People Learn: Brain, Mind, Experience, and School.*[11] Of special interest was a chapter devoted to *Expertise,* which said that "Experts have acquired extensive knowledge in their domain, but what distinguishes them most from novices is that their knowledge is organized along core concepts or principles, and they have an ability to look at a new situation and to see features and patterns not evident to the novice. Despite holding a vast repertoire of knowledge in their domain, that knowledge is conditioned so it can be selected, recalled, and applied in a seemingly effortless manner."

Experts demonstrate at least two other characteristics that differentiate them from novices. One of these is *metacognition*: they think about what they are learning, they make sense out of new information, they assess what they know and what they do not know, and they monitor what works and what does not in the application of their thinking.[11,12,13] These processes not only reinforce useful knowledge, they facilitate another characteristic of experts, namely their ability to *transfer* knowledge learned in one context to other contexts. As a result, experts are able to create useful new solutions to problems.

Gene Stead was an expert. However these comments about expertise tell us more than just the descriptors of an expert; they also tell us something important about how an expert's mind works. They get at the heart of how Gene Stead's brain worked and what made him so special.

He Liked Working with His Head

Gene said this: "[In Boston] I first learned that just as many people like to fish or play golf, I like to work with my head."[14] Actually that statement was an early insight about himself, which he later attributed to interacting with Soma Weiss, his most cherished mentor in Boston. Here is another arrangement of "Steadisms" quoted or paraphrased, and gathered together to illustrate how he worked with his head:

> The learning process can be divided into the accumulation of bits of information (memory), and the movement of these bits into patterns, which are new to the individual (thinking). Learning takes energy. The physician knows that all forms of learning require changes in the structure of the nervous system and, because a person both learns and forgets, it is obvious that many of these changes are reversible.[15] Problem solving may or may not involve thinking. If you read another person's solution to a problem, the answer is acquired through memory. On the other hand, solution of a problem by

the rearrangement of bits of information into patterns that are new to the individual is, by definition, thinking. Thinking takes time and it frequently serves as a stimulus to accumulate new bits of information.[16] Experienced doctors have firmly fixed in their minds a series of patterns, which covers all common illnesses. They quickly identify which pattern to call up as data from the history, physical examination, laboratory and special examinations come in.[17] Keep a store of well-worked and useful knowledge. Differentiate between the things that you know but can't be used by you in the middle of the night, and the things that you both know and use. Continually increase the usable material by finding ways to put known but non-used material to work.[18] One learns by asking oneself questions, then going out and finding the answers. If I am going to change my opinion I've at least got to know the basis for changing.[19]

How His Head Worked

In the 1930s, when Gene Stead was first observing how his own brain worked, psychologists appreciated the distinction between short-term, long-term, and working memory; understanding memory at a scientific level came later. Learning is a word now used to represent the process by which we acquire information about the world, while memory is a word used to represent the processes by which we store that information for retrieval at a later time. Memories are formed in stages. The first stage, *encoding*, requires a brief but adequate time period during which attention is focused on a sensory input and thereby activates an existing network of neuronal groups. Repeated activation of that network within a short time frame leads to facilitation of synaptic transmission, and the memory persists for seconds or minutes after the input is removed. This facilitated synaptic transmission represents the second stage of memory formation, so-called *short-term memory*. The conversion of short-term into long-term memories is referred to as *consolida-*

tion. This process involves gene expression, new protein synthesis, and the turnover of dendritic spines to produce long-term memories that last for hours, days, years, or even a lifetime.[20] That is what Gene Stead was referring to when he said, "learning requires energy" and changes brain structure.[21]

We are all familiar with the useful distinction between data and information. It is helpful in thinking about how the brain works to draw a parallel distinction between memory and knowledge. Knowledge depends on individual long-term memories that have been categorized as to their accuracy and importance. Knowledge also involves associations, connected maps of individual memories that are both accurate and related.[22,23] *Constructivism,* a theory articulated by educational psychologists, considers new knowledge to be built from what one already knows as a consequence of adding, subtracting, or correcting elements essential to understanding.[24] There are three messages from these considerations: First, knowledge (and by extrapolation expertise) are higher order cognitive capacities that depend upon poly-modal associative neural connections related to memory. Second, the learner actively builds those neural connections into structure. And third, the process of adding to or modifying existing knowledge is called thinking.

Gene Stead thought clearly about how his head worked. He not only used brain mechanisms, he was remarkably aware of the processes involved, and of the relevance of those processes to how others learned. He was a cognitive neuroscientist before that term was ever coined.

Brain Sorting

Gene Stead was fascinated with learning as a process, but he also was intrigued by differences among individuals. Indeed, he was much more interested in their differences than their similarities. His focus was on the implication that different nervous systems determine the different ways in which individual patients respond to a given disease. He also concentrated on how individuals learn in different ways, and even how those differences should guide career choices. Here again is Dr. Stead:

No two men are really ever alike.[25] The brain is our most complex organ and therefore brains can be expected to be more different from each other than are hearts or livers.[26] A large part of the structure of the brain is genetically determined, but environment and use of the system can greatly modify the mature system.[27] The physician knows that all purposeful behavior, which he observes in patients, is channeled through the nervous system.[15] Just as diseases can be sorted ... the brains of persons with diseases can be sorted.[28] The student should be taught to use behavior as a means of identifying structural similarities and dissimilarities among patients.[29] Students, interns, and residents come to us for training, but like patients each of them is different, and each gains satisfaction in a different way. Rather than trying to stamp out products in a single mold, I try to determine the best fit in life by helping a large number of students and residents work out their career pattern. Our goal is to identify the best use of the man and to find the limits imposed by his structure.[4] I was fortunate in having a clinical and laboratory apprenticeship under Soma Weiss, one of the great clinicians of the 1930s. Dr. Weiss was aware of the importance of the nervous system in regulating behavior. From that time on I was interested in what I call brain sorting.[30]

Why Brains Differ

Genetic instructions control the expression of proteins responsible for basic cellular functions, including differentiation of precursor cells into neurons, their growth and migration, the formation of synapses, and synaptic attributes such as excitability and the formation and release of specific neurotransmitters. However, the overall structural result is characterized as much by individual variability as by similarity. Even before birth, brain development has many epigenetic components. The brain's topology and the formation of specific neural groups and networks are not completely pre-specified by a genetic blueprint, but arise in part because of regional competition among neurons for growth factors, what Gerald Edelman calls *Neuronal Group Selection or Neural Darwinism.*[31,32] At another level, and largely after birth, synaptic connections within and between neurons can be strengthened or weakened based on use. Entire neuronal groups may disappear in the absence of use, and still others become connected as a result of experiences with the outside world. This has been referred to as *Experiential Selection.* These connections too are either made or enhanced by use. "No two men are ever really alike"[33] because no two brains develop in the same way. Gene Stead also said:

> If a hundred people listen to Beethoven, some will be in
> ecstasy and some will be bored. Some people lack a
> sense of direction or an appreciation for shapes. Other
> people are tune deaf, or color blind, or dyslexic. These
> are not good and bad people, but people with different
> central nervous systems.[34] The ability to make high
> grades in school and excel on aptitude tests may not
> translate into outstanding performance ... performance
> is greatly modified by non-IQ portions of our brains.[35]

In 1983, Howard Gardner challenged the long-held view that intelligence is a general intellectual capacity; possessed in varying degrees by everyone, measurable by a pencil and paper test, and reducible to a single number—the I.Q. In his book, *Frames of Mind,*[36] Gardner introduced a new view of intellectual capacity, which he called "Multiple Intelligences." Gardner started with the premise that "an intelligence is an intellectual competence that results either in the creation of a novel product or the solution of a problem," and he suggested criteria that could determine whether a candidate-ability should be regarded as an intelligence or not. His first criterion asserts that an intellectual competence can be either selectively destroyed or spared (ie, isolated) by brain injury. A closely related criterion states that a competence can be expressed in a precocious manner in otherwise normal children, or it can be present despite highly retarded performance in most or all other

intellectual domains (eg, the *idiot savant*). Furthermore, a competence, to be considered, must have plausible evolutionary antecedents
in other species (eg, language and bird songs). The seven or eight
competencies that Gardner classifies as "intelligences" meet several
of these criteria, and he concludes that each of them must be thought
of as one *intellectual potential* among several. According to Gardner these independent, neural-based, intellectual competencies are
comprised of the linguistic, musical, logical-mathematical, spatial,
bodily-kinesthetic, and personal intelligences (the latter embracing both a sense of self and separately a sense of others). A few of
the most notable features of Gardner's thoughts about "Multiple
Intelligences" are these: First, we all possess these intelligences and
perhaps more. Second, as a result of interactions between hered-
ity and environment during brain development, no two individuals express these intelligences in exactly the same proportion; rather,
we each have a unique profile of intellectual competencies and a
unique potential for their individual development. Finally, Gardner believes that properly structured assessments can identify relative strengths or weaknesses in each of the intellectual domains.

Before he died, I spoke with Gene Stead about Gardner's book
and about Gardner's thoughts: Gene viewed Gardner's ideas as another way to sort brains. He embraced the concept of multiple intellectual competencies, each expressed differently in any person.
He also viewed Gardner's thoughts as supportive of his (Stead's)
own idea that a teacher's role is not only to recognize within individuals where learning is easy and where it is hard, but to use that
information to identify the best use of the individual in the medical profession. What an extraordinary commitment by a teacher to
his students!

A Final Thought on Brain Differences: Communication

I get up (each morning) to communicate and learn.[37]
Effective communication requires that the doctor be

aware of wide differences in brain anatomy and the effects of those differences on the behavior of patients. Each doctor's brain also is unique, and the doctor has to understand that the pictures he or she is perceiving, and his or her views of reality and fantasy, differ from those of every other human being.[38] If I want to communicate with you, I have to have some way to form pictures in my mind and send them to you. In turn I must have the means to reconstruct pictures in my mind from material you send to me. The only way to evaluate the communication that actually occurred is for you to sketch out the material you have received and for me to sketch out the material I have sent. If the brains of sender and receiver were anatomically identical, there would be no problems in communication.[38] The mistake made by the young teacher is in thinking that the student is receiving, grasping, and learning all that is presented. This error in thinking is corrected by hearing the playback.[2]

Gene was very much aware of the complexities of communication between any two individuals, including doctor and patient or teacher and learner. Again, he attributed these difficulties to brain differences and to differences in how two brains process incoming information. Getting the receiver to play back what he or she has heard or learned, and then getting the sender to provide feedback is the best solution to this dilemma. What a marvelous illustration of his genuine interest in patients and learners!

Computers Will Change Medicine

Gene understood that memories not used are forgotten or sometimes recalled in distorted ways.[39] In 1967, he pushed several of us at Duke (with the help of NIH) to acquire a digital computer and to build what he called a "New Textbook of Medicine". It was to be a digital record of all of our patients, with initial descriptors, treatments undertaken, and outcomes over time. He was convinced that no one could really remember all their patients, select those most similar to the current patient, or apply statistically valid approaches to predict outcomes with treatments A or B or C. He anticipated that a computer would be far better at such tasks. Our initial effort was focused on patients with myocardial infarction and later broadened to become the Duke Cardiology Database. Later still it was expanded further to include other conditions and data from other institutions.

Gene's early concept was to use computers to correct an inherent deficit in human memory. Much later (probably in the late 1990s) he began to use and experience the Internet. And in his maverick way he said: "why should students memorize anything they will soon forget if they can learn to look it up when they need it with a search engine on the Internet."[40] By then Gene's idea had *morphed*, from simply expanding human memory through computers into substituting connected computers for human memory. This would free up "brain time" for thinking, which he regarded as a higher order cognitive function for which brains were better suited. In some ways Gene Stead's use of experience in medicine was analogous to Vannevar Bush's use of technology to deal with the challenge of exponential growth in human knowledge. In his 1945 essay *As We May Think*.[41] Bush envisioned "the personal computer … voice recognition software, hypertext, and even the World Wide Web." In a short introduction to that essay the editor notes that Bush is now widely regarded as providing the "early road map to the Internet age." Gene Stead's ideas about computers and medicine may prove to be comparably clairvoyant.

Optimal Learning Environments

The 1998 NRC report, *How People Learn*[11] summarized much of what I have tried to highlight in this essay, and more. The report's authors list several ideas central to the connection between emerging brain science and learning: no two individuals are identical; experience changes brain structure; changes in structure have functional consequences; and different parts of the brain learn at different times. A further example of such connection was their emphasis that usable knowledge consists not just of facts stored in memory, but of information that is organized in ways that contribute to an applicable understanding. *How People Learn* can be viewed as a synthesis of brain development—how the brain learns and the functional characteristics of memory, knowledge, thinking, multiple intelligences, and the convergence of these concepts in the forms of understanding and expertise. Flowing from that synthesis was a conclusion: "Optimal learning environments are *purposefully* created" and they have the following characteristics:

- They start by acquiring insights into what people bring to the setting in terms of pre-existing knowledge, relevant prior experiences, significant culture beliefs about the domain, and the motivation to learn. *They are learner-centered!*
- They focus on elements known to promote initial learning: motivation, attention, practice, adequate time, how incomplete knowledge or errors of fact can bias new understanding, the organization and clustering of information around concepts and principles, and the provision of examples of transferability. *They are knowledge-centered!*
- They focus on need for a learner's knowledge and understanding to be made visible, either in verbal or written form, and then used as a basis for formative feedback. *They are assessment-centered!*
- They emphasize that a learner's thinking should be shared: with teachers, with other learners, with family, and with individuals including experts in a knowledge-based community. These activities involve practice at more than one level, but of equal importance they help to establish what cultural norms are and the extent to which the learner's thinking is valued. *They are community-centered!*

I am astounded at how Gene Stead purposefully created, in the 1940s and 50s, an environment for learning medicine that matched so well what was described fifty years later as "optimal." Gene would have added a fifth element to the optimal learning environment—a computer with a large memory and a good search engine!

Stead's Legacy

Dr. Stead was a gifted teacher and he made a huge difference. Another like him is not likely to come along. Even if he could be cloned, one of the messages in this essay is that the copy would not have a brain identical to his. So the best we can do is capture and articulate his legacy.

Dr. Stead's legacy begins with his conviction that in any educational institution the *primary* product is molded and trained men and women. That is the highest priority of a medical school, and a conscious commitment to that purpose is essential. Gene was an expert, but he recognized that "effective teaching is a skill associated with, but separate from content expertise."[42] He did not dismiss the importance of teachers or of teaching, but his emphasis was on learners and learning. By observing how he himself learned, how others learned, and how his mentors had promoted learning environments, he developed a remarkable insight into how brains work. He applied his insights about cognition and learning theory to learning at all levels. He recognized that no two people were ever alike, that they came to any situation with different experiences, different ways of learning, different aptitudes, and they found satisfactions from work in different ways. He didn't just tolerate those differences; he viewed finding the best use for each individual as his responsibility. At teaching rounds or clinical conferences Gene insisted that the patient be physically present. The patient and solving his or her problem was the best motive to learn. The fact that no two people are alike was as true of patients as it was of learners, so he wanted to see the person with the disease, not just hear about the disease. And, he didn't want to render an opinion or advice without seeing the patient and making his own observations. Gene taught attitudes, attitudes like constant awareness of the distinction between what you know and what you don't know, that you learn by asking questions and finding answers, and that you learn most when you teach. He taught pattern recognition rather than diagnosis, that what you do is important but why you do it is even more important, and that finding your own way to derive satisfaction with medicine was essential. As a departmental chair at Duke, Gene served on the admissions committee, he taught physical diagnosis, he conducted teaching rounds eleven months each year, he took morning report with second year residents and the chief resident, and he regularly attended "Sunday School," the weekly conference where residents picked a topic that interested them, read about it in the library, and presented what they had learned. Gene was deeply interested in the people who trained with him and he spent extended time with them. He realized that it took time, not only to "groove their nervous systems" but also to evaluate their growth potential. Because they were the principal product of his educational system, one-time or only occasional interactions with learners were simply insufficient to his purpose.

I have enjoyed reflecting on Dr. Stead and trying to capture and articulate his legacy. But the purpose of this effort is not to write an essay. Rather, it is to pass his legacy on to others. Gene Stead was very special and ahead of his time. He communicated messages of fundamental importance. Those messages have been reinforced by what has been learned subsequently about brain science, about learning, and about optimal learning environments. Those fundamental messages need reaffirmation and purposeful incorporation into the learning environments we call medical schools.[42] Medical schools have changed, but the development of people who are the primary products of our medical schools continues. It is simply too important a purpose to leave to chance!

References

1. Wagner GS, Cebe B, Rozear MP. (Eds). E.A. Stead Jr. *What This Patient Needs is a Doctor*. Durham, NC. Carolina Academic Press; 1978.

2. Stead EA Jr. *Just Say For Me*. Schoonmaker F, Metz E (eds). Denver, CO. World Press, Inc. 1968.

3. Stead EA Jr. *A Way of Thinking: A Primer on Being a Doctor*. Haynes BF (ed). Durham, N.C.: Carolina Academic Press; 1995. p.10.

4. Wagner, G. Op.cit. p.32.

5. Ibid. p.3.

6. Ibid. p.68.

7. Stead 1968. Op.cit. p.59.

8. Wagner, G. Op.cit. p.67.

9. Stead 1968. Op.cit. p.62.

10. Laszlo J, Neelon FA. *The Doctors' Doctor: A Biography of Eugene A. Stead Jr., MD.* Durham, NC: Carolina Academic Press; 2006.

11. Brunsford JD, Brown AL, Cocking RR. (Eds.). *How People Learn: Brain, Mind, Experience, and School.* Washington, D.C.: National Academy Press, 1999.

12. Flavell, JH. Metacognition and Cognitive Monitoring: A New Area of Cognitive-Developmental Inquiry. Am Psychol. 1979: 34(10): 906–911.

13. Livingston JA. Metacognition: An Overview. 1997. Web site: http://www.gse.buffalo.edu/fas/shuell/CEP564/Metacog.htm. Accessed February 20, 2008.

14. Stead 1968. Op.cit. p.77.

15. Wagner, G. Op.cit. p.66.

16. Stead 1995. Op.cit. p.19–20.

17. Ibid. p.21.

18. Wagner, G. Op.cit. p.7.

19. Stead 1968. Op.cit. p.50.

20. Kandel ER, Schwartz JH, Jessell TM. *Principles of Neuro Science.* 4th Ed. New York, NY: McGraw-Hill, Inc; 2000.

21. Stead 1968. Op.cit. p.52.

22. Bressler SL. Understanding Cognition Through Large-Scale Cortical Networks. Curr Dir Psychol Sc. 2002;11:58–61.

23. Bruner, JS. *Contemporary Approaches to Cognition. Cambridge, MA: Harvard University Press.* [Reprinted in Bruner, J.S. *Going Beyond the Information Given.* New York: Norton Press. 1973: pp.218–22].

24. Bruner JS. Constructivist Theory. 2001. Web site: http://tip.psychology.org/bruner.html. Accessed February 20, 2008.

25. Stead 1968. Op.cit. p.15.

26. Stead 1995. Op.cit. p.17.

27. Ibid. p.101.

28. Ibid. p.97.

29. Stead 1968. Op.cit. p.48.

30. Stead 1995. Op.cit. p.106.

31. Edelman GM. *Neural Darwinism: The Theory of Neuronal Group Selection.* NY: Basic Books. 1987.

32. Edelman GM. *Bright Air, Brilliant Fire: On the Matter of the Mind.* New York, NY: Basic Books. 1992.

33. Stead 1968. Op.cit. p.15.

34. Ibid. p.16.

35. Stead 1996. Op.cit. p.108.

36. Gardner H. *Frames of Mind: The Theory of Multiple Intelligences.* 2nd Ed. New York, NY: Basic Books: A Member of The Perseus Books Company. 1993.

37. Stead 1968. Op.cit. p.51.

38. Stead 1995. Op.cit. p.15.

39. Schacter DL. *The Seven Sins of Memory: How the Mind Forgets and Remembers.* Boston, MA: Hough Mifflin Company. 2001.

40. Stead, EA Jr., Starmer, F. Google and the Internet: Is Life-Long Memorization Any Longer Necessary. 2003. Web site. http://easteadjr.org/thoughts.html. (See Mostly My Thoughts: Thoughts About Learning). Accessed April 28, 2008.

41. Bush, V. As We May Think. Atlantic Monthly, July 1945. [Reprinted in: *The American Idea: The Best of Atlantic Monthly.*] Doubleday, A Division of Random House Inc., New York, NY; 2007. pp.78–83].

42. Wilkerson L, Irby DM. Strategies for Improving Teaching Practices: A Comprehensive Approach to Faculty Development. Acad Med. 1998;73(4):387–96.

Chapter 2

The Patient Is the
Focus of Doctoring

Francis A. Neelon, MD

When Eugene Stead came to make attending rounds on Osler Ward, he often began the session with a brief account of some aspect of "Medicine" that had been on his mind. Oftentimes he would postulate about the state of the world, or science, or how doctors were affecting—or being affected by either. His ramblings were not uninteresting, but they seemed abstract and distant from the hurly-burly of clinical medicine with which the students and house staff were struggling. We were champing at the bit to discuss the last night's admissions, to demonstrate to the professor our diagnostic skills and therapeutic savvy. We were always pleased when he turned from the ethereal to the practical and said: "Who do we have to see?"

Three or four or more patients would have been admitted during the preceding day, and on Stead's signal we would troop to a patient's bed, where the student or intern would recount the patient's story and the details of the exam. Occasionally, a recently admitted patient was not physically present on the ward, having been sent off the floor for diagnostic studies or surgery (or perhaps to the morgue). We couldn't wait to tell him about these "fascinating cases," and to discuss the disease processes that had led to admission. He would have none of that. He told me that talking about disease in the absence of the sick individual herself, was "dry rounds"; they didn't interest him. We were already so excited about our medical prowess, about what we had seen and done and thought about in these cases, that Stead felt his job here was already done. He would, I suspect, have agreed with William Osler who cited John Locke's admonition that when teachers "give a pupil 'a relish of knowledge' [they] put life into his work."[1] Stead saw his job as infusing relish into us already jaded young medicos by making us consider patients still on the ward, even when they seemed to us less "interesting" or medically exciting.

Stead's technique was encapsulated in Dr. Bob Whalen's account of his time on Osler Ward:

> [As medical residents] we wanted to treat "real" diseases, not neurotic complaints. In our opinion Mrs. A was floridly "psychoneurotic" and there was nothing we could do for her. We knew, though, that we would be in high hot water if Stead ever got to round on this woman. He would spend all day asking us questions about her and her life that we wouldn't be able to answer because no one had taken the time to really go over her case. We hid her on the back porch of the old Osler Ward, hoping he'd never find her, and for a short time we deluded ourselves into thinking we could get away with it. He had a nose for trouble though, and on gallop rounds, which were apt to last for 4 to 5 hours as he checked on every patient, he found her. He spent an hour and a half at the bedside of this lady as all of us developed varicose veins trying to answer his questions. Thereafter he made a point of stopping by everyday to check on her ... he even stopped by Osler Ward during his vacation when he came in to pick up his mail. When it was time for her release, I held my breath as Stead asked, "Now who's going to follow Mrs. A in the clinic?" Obviously, there were no volunteers, but since I was the resident, Stead gave me the honor, though ... I really couldn't understand why he thought this patient's case was so important. In fact, it puzzled me that he would make such an effort to see that she got the best care when we had patients with much more serious ill-

nesses. Dr. Stead's teaching was remarkable that way. He often didn't explain why he thought something was important for you to know; he presumed you'd figure it out somewhere along the line. . . .

Four or five years later, . . . I asked Dr. Stead why he insisted that we be so involved with Mrs. A. He told me he figured this woman had a large family structure that would have been destroyed if she became really incapacitated. She had a child who suffered from diabetes insipidus and had to have her fluids carefully regulated with pituitary hormone, and her husband was working at graduating from school at the time. If she were completely unable to function, her daughter and husband would have suffered severely as well. As it turned out, I did follow her and have for over 30 years. True, she has had a lot of ups and downs, but she has managed to remain functional, which clearly made a critical difference in all their lives. Her husband earned a degree in political science and went on to become Chairman of the Department of Political Science at a university. Stead never said, "If you can keep this woman going for 25 or 30 years, you're going to keep her daughter going and her husband functional." He never spelled things out that clearly, but usually the lesson eventually came home — some of us were just slow learners.[2]

Stead was equally insistent that patients be physically present at Grand Rounds. Every week at Duke and at the Veteran's Administration Hospital across the street, two faculty members discussed the cases of two patients who were in the hospital at the time, and who came to the amphitheater as their case history was recounted. After a few questions, the patient returned to the ward, and the discussion began, focused at least by implication on the patient's illness. At times we wondered why we bothered having the patient there at all; just have the speaker launch right in and save time for dispensing "information." Alas, we must be careful what we wish for, because that is what has happened. As Howard Spiro points out, the focus of Grand Rounds has shifted "from a patient to a case [so that] less and less time [is] allowed for talking to the patient, until he [has become] an icon of himself, a case, present like the American flag to show that there was a patient/person somewhere in the background."[3] But Stead (and later Jim Wyngaarden) insisted that patients remain present as the focal point of Grand Rounds.

After Stead had stepped down as chairman, I once called to ask if he would speak at Grand Rounds. "No," he told me (and my heart sank), "but I will lead the discussion." I think that captures the essence of his view: Grand Rounds was not the place to lecture about the abstraction of "disease" but was the place to contemplate the singularities of one individual who happened to carry the burden of this or that disease. Concepts of disease are important but only in the context of the specific sick patient. By having the patient always present, the central focus of medicine (the care of the sick) need not be overtly noted—it is bred in the bone.

A Brief Historical Excursion

The patient has not always been the focus of medical education—and even when that idea was honored, the honor generally did not last, a condition that persists to the present. Formal medical education in medieval Europe consisted of lectures delivered by a professor reciting the theories of Galen (AD 129–200), followed perhaps by a brief period of apprenticeship with a practitioner (informal medical education provided only the apprenticeship and dispensed with lectures). Things changed in 1537, when the 23 year-old Andreas Vesalius was appointed to the faculty of medicine at Padua and began the anatomical studies that culminated in his great text, *De Humani Corporis Fabrica* (On the Fabric of the Human Body). Vesalius was the first professor to come down from the lecture podium and take the dissecting scalpel in hand, and thus uncovered numerous errors in the anatomical teaching of Galen, which had been based on animal anatomy. In the intellectual ferment that ensued, Giovanni Battista da Monte (Montanus) began to take his pupils out of the lecture hall and into the nearby hospital of Saint Francis where he taught them at the bedsides of his patients. Padua became the center of the medical world.

But this happy state did not last. After da Monte's death in 1551, medical teaching returned to its prior, lecture-only format, and clinical education languished. By 1600, Padua had resumed its status as a *scola de pulsibus et urinus* (a school of pulse [counting] and urine [inspection]). As Osler pointed out, the Temple of Minerva Medica is not fixed, but portable; the center of the medical universe stays in one location for 50 or 100 years, then moves on. By 1650, Leiden had become the centerpoint, largely because Franciscus Sylvius successfully initiated the practice of bedside teaching there ("I led my students by the hand to the practice of medicine, taking them every day to see patients in the public hospital"). After Sylvius, Hermann Boerhaave continued bedside teaching, but after his death, it again faltered, and Minerva moved her temple to Edinburgh, from which academic medicine came to the American colonies. It is possible to follow the peregrinations of Minerva across Europe and eventually to the US, but I don't wish to belabor the point, only to emphasize that in each instance the flourishing of medicine was accompanied by an intense and gyroscopic focus on the patient. It is not possible to prove that the one causes the other, but I do not doubt the connection.

The Arid Landscape of 21st Century Clinical Teaching

It is possible to trace backwards the influences of medical teaching on a given individual and thereby construct a "medical" genealogy of that person.[4] Take, for example, Eugene Stead; it is not surprising that he carried proudly the banner of bedside instruction. Stead gave credit for this to Soma Weiss, who had brought him from Cincinnati to the Thorndike Lab. Weiss, in turn had been recruited by Francis Peabody, whose early mentors were Joseph Pratt and William Thayer, both of whom had long periods of tutelage under William Osler. It is possible to discern further sources of

Osler's inspiration,[5] but for our purposes it is enough to trace Stead's forebears back to this sentinel figure whose, devotion to the idea of bedside teaching was so strong that he said he wanted his obituary to read only that "I taught students in the wards."[6,7] Osler further said "it is a safe rule to have no teaching without a patient for a text, and the best teaching is that taught by the patient himself."[8] So it is not hard to see how Stead came by the idea that the physical presence of the patient is central to any clinical teaching exercise (of course, Stead would have called these learning, not teaching, exercises) — to see how the baton was passed, hand by hand, from Osler to Pratt and Thayer to Peabody to Weiss to Stead. What has happened since?

All the evidence says that we have let the baton slip through our fingers. Thirty years ago, Eugene Linfors and I were struck by the fact that medical students coming to Duke to interview for internship positions returned from a visit on teaching rounds saying that they had never before seen patients' cases presented or discussed at the bedside.[9] Reports since then confirm what our student applicants said: bedside teaching has nearly disappeared from view.[10–12] Direct observations[13–15] show that 10% or less of the time devoted to "rounds" is spent in the presence of the patient; most of the time is spent in a classroom where a chalkboard and x-ray viewbox are available and the teacher can assume the role of "talking book," giving a mini-lecture to a group of comfortably seated — and passive — listeners (who promptly forget almost everything the teacher tells them[15]). Not surprisingly under those circumstances, students value most those teachers who can talk spontaneously on a great variety of medical topics. This situation is vastly different from the teaching atmosphere engendered by Eugene Stead, who steadfastly *refused* to give treatment advice except to point out where or from whom the desired information could be obtained. Rather than dole out specifics — info poured from the full vessel of the teacher into the empty vessel of the student — Stead sought to "create a shadowy framework in which the student can climb."[16] Stead knew what most of the world never learned or had forgotten — that the "effectiveness of the teacher must be judged by the things that happen after the student and teacher part company,"[16] not by the transitory phenomenon of the "teaching" moment.

Can We Water the Desert?

The word "clinical" comes through Latin from the Greek "*klinikos*" meaning "pertaining to the sick-bed." Given this etymology, it is surprising to find that a mere 10–20% of the time nominally devoted to clinical teaching is actually spent at the bedside of the sick person.[17] Stead never let rounds drift from the bedside, even when there was (so we thought) good reason for such a translocation. Today, just 40 years after Stead gave up the reins as chairman, the whole of medical education has lost touch with the *genius loci* of the bedside. How has this happened?

Table 1 lists some of the factors that tend to drive learners away from the bedside. There is little doubt that Item 1 reflects the imposition of strict duty hours for house offices and the drying up of revenue sources to pay the attending physician; the summed result is an evaporation of the unencumbered time needed for teaching and learning—to the point that just the time needed to traipse to the bedside can seem an unaffordable luxury. It will take real effort

Table 1. Excuses for Not Going to the Bedside

1. There is "not enough time" to do everything
2. Comfort of the participants (seating; coffee)
3. Availability of paraphernalia (chalkboard, viewbox, charts)
4. A desire to protect the "privacy" of the patient
5. A fear that the patient will dislike hearing his case recounted aloud
6. The patient won't be in the bed anyway
7. The professor can control content and direction of the discussion
8. Learners can avoid the risk of public embarrassment
9. Professors can avoid the risk of public embarrassment

and ingenuity by department chairs to overcome these forces. Items 2 and 3 relate to learner preferences and are not insuperable obstacles. Items 4 and 5 are often cited as reasons to avoid the bedside but these have been largely disproved by evaluations of patients after beside rounds.[9,12,18,19] Item 6 is a bona-fide problem that reflects the accelerated pace of hospitalization; being sure that the patient will not be off the floor for some diagnostic or therapeutic procedure requires concerted effort by hospital administration and the resident in charge of the rounds.

There is no way to be sure, but my guess is that, apart from item 1, items 7–9 are the major forces distracting teachers and learners from the bedside. Professors who see themselves as "talking books," capable of delivering erudite mini-lectures on several (but certainly not all) medical topics, fear that a trip to the bedside will set them skating on the thin-ice of their competence, if not completely under the water of ignorance. They and the students with them all want to avoid the loss of face that comes from public revelation of incompetence or ineptitude. This is nothing new: in 1636 when Otto van Heurne of Leyden first proposed to question students in the presence of patients, he was forced to withdraw his proposal because "that style displeased most of [the students]."[20] As van Huerne's successor, Sylvius, successfully demonstrated,[9] those resistances can be overcome if the teacher correctly visualizes his or her role as a questioner rather than an answerer,[21] and if he or she insist that students come with them to the bedside.[10,11]

There are many benefits from insisting, as Stead always did, that we make the patient the focus of our clinical gaze. As Aristotle implies, an artist can be an artist even if he keeps all the pictures he paints out of sight in the attic, and a poet can be a poet even if she keeps all her writings secreted in a drawer; but a farmer cannot be a farmer unless he plants a garden, and only if he has a patient, is a doctor a doctor. In Table 2, I have compiled a list of some of the benefits of focusing on the patient, but they all boil down to a conception of the doctor's job that sees beyond clinical physiology and pharmacology to the ultimate goal of doc-

Table 2. Reasons to Go to the Bedside

1. The patient is seen as a real, living, breathing, *human* being
2. The patient can be made part of the dynamic of care
3. The skills of human interaction can be modeled
4. The skills of clinical examination can put on display
5. The teaching ("doctoring") role of doctors is made explicit
6. Pupils and teacher are on equal footing as "students" at the bedside
7. Because mysteries arise, curiosity is ascendant; questions supplant answers
8. All can see that "care of the patient" means more than "treatment of disease"

toring: how can we, with a knowledge of the science of body and mind, and a concern for the humanity of the patient, help this person in trouble.[22] Of course, if that is not your idea of the doctor's job, then the bedside will not be the place for you; if it is, there really is no other. To talk about "disease" is to talk about the ways in which 100 (or 1,000 or 10,000) different people are alike; to talk about "illness" is to talk about the ways in which the individual before us is unique in his manifestation of and response to disease. Over and over again, Stead's challenges to us came down to different ways of asking two questions: 1) How do we know what we think we know (about this patient? about medicine and science? about the world at large?). 2) What role can the doctor play in helping this patient get better?

Osler emphasized that the "whole art of medicine is in observation,"[23] and it is only at the bedside that we can hope to follow Yogi Berra's famous dictum: "You can observe a lot just by watching." To think about the "case" without the presence of the patient herself is to spin a fantasy of how things might be, is to devalue the very thing that makes medicine medicine—the tangible interaction of the doctor and the patient who has come for help.

Finale

At the end of rounds with Dr. Stead on Osler Ward, we would have seen the third or fourth of the previous day's admissions. Dr. Stead would have known nothing about any of the patients until we assembled at the bedside and the student or intern began the case presentation. After much give and take with and about the patient and the learners, we would go back to the doctors' office on Osler Ward to think about what had transpired. Often as not, the conversation would turn to the very points with which Stead had begun the session — now not some abstract and distant concept of little value to us laboring in the vineyard, but concrete and real, exemplified in the very case of the patient we had just seen together. It was magic — it was like pulling rabbits from a hat!

References

1. Osler W. "The Master Word in Medicine" in *Aequanimitas with Other Addresses*, 3rd ed. Philadelphia; P Blakiston's Son & Co. 1932.

2. Laszlo J, Neelon FA. *The Doctors' Doctor*. Durham, NC; Carolina Academic Press. 2006;p.203–4.

3. Spiro HM. *Doctors, Patients and Placebos*. New Haven; Yale University Press. 1986, p.72.

4. LaComb M. Taking a history. Harvard Medical Alumni Bulletin. 2005;78(3):24–31.

5. Bryan CS. The influence of Sir Andrew Clark (1826–1893) on William Osler (1849–1919). J Med Biogr. 2005;23:195–200.

6. Osler W. "The Fixed Period" in *Aequanimitas with Other Addresses*, 3rd ed. Philadelphia; P Blakiston's and Son. 1932.

7. Barondess JA. Is Osler dead? Perspect Biol Med. 2002;45:65–84.

8. Osler W. "The Hospital as a College" in *Aequanimitas with Other Addresses*, 3rd ed. Philadelphia; P Blakiston's Son & Co. 1932.

9. Linfors EW, Neelon FA. The case for bedside rounds. N Engl J Med 1980;303:1230–3.

10. Fitzgerald FT. Bedside teaching. West J Med. 1993;158:418–20.

·11. LaCombe MA. On bedside teaching. Ann Intern Med. 1997; 126:217–20.

12. Wang-Cheng RM, Barnas GP, Sigmann P, Riendl PA, Young MJ. Bedside case presentations: why patients like them but learners don't. J Gen Intern Med 1989;4:284–7.

13. Tremonti LP, Biddle WB. Teaching behaviors of residents and faculty members. J Med Ed. 1982; 57:854–9.

14. Miller M, Johnson B, Greene HL, Baier M, Nowlin S. An observational study of attending rounds. J Gen Intern Med. 1992;7:646–8.

15. Elliot DL, Hickam DH. Attending rounds on in-patient units: differences between medical and non-medical services. Med Educ. 1993;27:503–8.

16. Stead EA Jr. The limitations of teaching. Pharos. 1969;32:54–7.

17. Williams KN, Ramani S, Fraser B, Orlander JD. Improving bedside teaching: findings from a focus group study of learners. Acad Med. 2008; 83:257–64.

18. Simons RJ, Baily RG, Zelis R, Zwillich CW. The physiologic and psychological effects of the bedside presentation. N Eng. J Med. 1989;321:1273–5.

19. Lehmann LA, Brancati FL, Chen M-C, Roter D, Dobs, AS. The effect of bedside case presentations on patients' perceptions of their medical care. N Engl J Med. 1997;336:1150–5.

20. von Ziemssen H. Ueber den klinischen Unterricht in Deutschland. Dtsch Arch Klin Med. 1874;13:1–20.

21. Fitzgerald FT. Curiosity. Ann Intern Med. 1999;130:70–72.

22. Peabody FW. The care of the patient. JAMA 1927;88:877–82.

23. Belkin BM, Neelon FA. The Art of Observation: William Osler and the Method of Zadig. Ann Intern Med. 1992;1160:863–6.

Comments Following "The Patient Is the Focus of Doctoring"

William W. ("Bill") Stead, MD, Associate Vice Chancellor for Health Affairs, Chief Strategy and Information Officer, McKesson Foundation Professor of Biomedical Informatics and Professor of Medicine at Vanderbilt University Medical Center, grew up with Gene Stead, served as his intern, and "he and Mother were my wife's and my best friends through the early years of our marriage":

I think there are two aspects to focusing on the patient. One is the idea that the doctor or the clinician is the person who takes responsibility for the patient. Largely, we have lost the idea that one person is to take responsibility for the patient, to care about the patient as an individual. That missing piece, I at least believe, has led to the fragmentation of health care.

Another part of focusing on the patient is that you learn most in the direct presence of the patient. You've clearly got to observe and listen to the patient if you're going to take responsibility and truly understand and care about that individual. Just knowing the results of the patient's tests is not enough. I think increasingly that we need to put together other social and environmental information about the patient, which you may or may not be able to glean at the bedside. It all needs to be put together in a holistic picture. As best I can tell, we're not doing either at this moment.

Morton D. ("Mort") Bogdonoff, MD, Chief Resident under Stead in 1954–55 and now Emeritus Professor of Medicine at Weill Cornell College of Medicine, takes third-year medical students on bedside rounds five days a week in the format used during Gene Stead's tenure as chairman:

I think the issue really boils down to the fact that people keep saying there's no time to do what we're talking about — to actually go and see the patient. I'm still active in teaching at Cornell, and when I insist that we must be in the presence of the patient, they say to me, "Oh, Dr. Bogdonoff, the patient's down at nuclear medicine"; so I say, "Well let's go down there because we know the patient is just sitting in the waiting room" — and invariably that's the case.

I get all the teaching prizes nowadays because there is no competition. No one else does what we're talking about, and the reason they give is that they don't have time. Time is money, and there is not enough money, and that is the reason it's no longer done. Unless we reallocate our resources, I think we can admire Gene Stead for what he taught us, but it's awfully hard to get other people to do it now.

I also feel that Bill Stead's notion of responsibility is absolutely crucial. In our institution now, when the admitting physician is a community-based practitioner (all of whom, by the way, are quite seasoned and well-informed) it is *unlikely, unlikely,* that that doctor will ever meet with the resident taking care of the patient in the hospital—and certainly never with the students. When I tell the house officers to call up and arrange to see the admitting physician, they tell me they can't get through because the phones are answered by office guard dogs who bite very hard. It is extremely rare for the house staff to see the doctor who takes care of the patient outside the hospital.

Ruth Ballweg, MPA, PA-C, Associate Professor, Director of the Physician Assistant Program at the University of Washington, and Past-President of the Society for the Preservation of Physician Assistant History, first met Dr. Stead while serving as President for the Association of Physician Assistant Programs in 1990–91:

Being from the University of Washington, I am impressed with how Dr. Stead's teaching legacy has extended throughout the United States. It's fascinating to see that some of the best teachers leave a trail that traces back to Dr. Stead. That's something that I think really should be acknowledged because the problem we're talking about isn't just at Duke; it's really everywhere.

At the twenty-fifth anniversary celebration for the PA profession, Dr. Stead told me, "One of my hidden agendas was that I wanted to prove to my students and my residents that doctors aren't the only smart people, and that physician assistants and others can make a contribution." That really changed the culture because PAs and nurse practitioners were sometimes more comfortable talking about what they didn't know! That gets back to the question here: why are people uncomfortable teaching in front of patients? I think the whole litigious nature of our culture plays a part that hasn't been discussed yet. People are not comfortable talking in front of the patient about a wide range of possibilities—"it might be this … or this … or this." Getting comfortable saying that "We're working through things and we don't really know the answer" is one of the big issues.

Another problem is the focus on inpatient teaching when so much care today is ambulatory care. We need to think about how to convert the teaching model. How do medical teachers deal with students in an ambulatory setting compared to a hospital setting where they see patients for longer periods of time, where you can see illness evolve or treatment take effect? How do we make sure that primary care people are involved in teaching as well? Ambulatory care; primary care; making it safe; those important issues resonate with the messages that Dr. Stead passed on to us.

Jeffrey ("Jeff") Wong, MD, Senior Associate Dean for Medical Education at the Medical University of South Carolina, met Dr. Stead while serving as Assistant Professor of Medicine at Duke in the late 1980s-mid 1990s:

My brain is actually right now being changed by all of this discussion, and I recognize that a lot of the teachings that passed down to me from my mentors at Duke—Dr. Greenfield, Dr. Neelon, Dr. Silberman, Dr. Wagner, and others—obviously originated with Dr. Stead. Their "second-generation Steadisms" have come through loud and clear in my own education.

To talk directly to the question of the value of having the patient physically present: it strikes me that I often see teaching that is focused on disease, and when that is the focus, it's probably not necessary to have the patient there. From what I have gleaned about Dr. Stead, he wasn't interested in just the disease when he was on "thinking rounds." He wanted to talk about how to take care of the patient—a distinction that is very hard for many learners to grasp. As I understand things, Dr. Stead expected and demanded that people learn about disease on their own, but they needed the patient in the room to actually learn about taking care of a patient with the disease. That to me seems to be a very important distinction.

Just like Dr. Bogdonoff, I often find the patients gone when we come on teaching rounds—and not just there. Grand Rounds have morphed from what they were to what we have now. Several years ago I ran a Grand Rounds at Yale where we actually had the patient in the room! It was a case of West Nile Virus, presenting as post-polio syndrome. The woman that we took care of was there in front of the room, and the whole dynamic was absolutely unlike any of other Grand Rounds in my six years at Yale. It was remarkable to see that difference—enough so that I'd say it's always valuable to have the patient present.

Harold Reiter ("Hal") Silberman, MD, currently Emeritus Professor of Medicine at Duke, served as Chief Resident at the Durham VA Hospital under Harvey Estes and, influenced by Gene Stead, managed to adjust his careers in medicine 6 times before becoming a medical/legal and insurance consultant after retiring for the third time:

I suggest that we think about the value of this process to the professor. If the professor is to evaluate the learner, how could he or she possibly do it without having touched the patient, reviewed the history and the physical exam? In the absence of the patient I can tell whether my learner is in touch with reality or not, or whether what he's telling me makes sense or not, but I can't determine whether his observations are actually correct or not. It's a very simple answer to the question about why it helps the teacher to have the patient present; other answers might look at why rounds are valuable to the patient.

Charles ("Chuck") Beauchamp, MD, PhD, is presently the only internist in a rural and poor county of 40,000 where he also serves as an instructor in "Public Health Biology" for students in the local Early College High School; he first met Eugene Stead in 1967 when he was a second year student on Long Ward and Stead was one of the two attending physicians:

A number of settings could further Dr. Stead's approach to teaching. One is the Veterans' Administration Hospital where there are opportunities to continue to do what Dr. Stead did: connect with the primary care physician of the patient. Another is the Fremont Free Clinic where, in that rural environment, there are only you, the patient and the students. Without all the accouterments of the hospital, you can continue the tradition of learning together from the patient. And a third setting is all the way out into the community, the home of the patient. That takes time, but in that setting you do incorporate the physical and socioeconomic surroundings of the patient, and the family.

Francis A. ("Frank") Neelon, MD, served as intern under Eugene Stead and later was Stead's associate editor at the North Carolina Medical Journal; after 40 years on the Duke faculty, he retired to become Medical Director of the Rice Diet Program:

Just to clarify a point, I'm not sure that our VA looks any different from Duke Hospital. Do you think teaching at the VA is somehow different from teaching at the university hospital?

Chuck Beauchamp: Well, a number of times the house staff there have contacted me as primary care physician of the patient. They would run by their questions about my care of the patient, and the process of discharge and transfer back to me. I just feel comfortable with that environment. I think that the VA has an economic scenario that's a little bit different from Duke Hospital in terms of how long the patient stays there, and the medico-legal aspects of interacting with the patient.

Harvey Jay Cohen, MD, Chairman of the Department of Medicine at Duke and Director, Center for the Study of Aging and Human Development, served as intern and resident under Eugene Stead, and later became his "boss" (Stead's words) when Stead "helped me start the Geriatrics Program" at the VA Hospital:

I want to follow up specifically on that point. I would disagree with the idea that the VA is not different from Duke Hospital. When I took on the Chairmanship [of Duke's Department of Medicine], I elected to continue to round at the VA rather than shift over to Duke, and I did that for a few reasons. One of them is that on the general medicine service at Duke there is tremendous pressure to move patients quickly through the system, and while patients are often seen by the attending physicians and house staff together, it is a very evanescent interaction — very quick and not sustained very much — simply because of lack of time. The VA *is* different. There is more time and less economic pressure. When I round, I insist as Eugene Stead did, that we see every patient in person, and we sometimes trail down to radiology or dialysis to see them there.

I tell the house staff they're looking in the wrong place if they expect me to list every antibiotic to be used for every bizarre infectious disease that we might happen to see. I can tell them which infectious disease consultant to call, but I'm not going to answer that question. What I can answer is: is this patient sick? how do we need to think about him? what are the ways we can think about him? how can we get to an answer about what's going on? how do these questions fit into the broader context of the patient? In my view, those questions can only be posed to the learners when we're seeing the patient together at the bedside. It's important that a fair percentage of the attending physicians at the VA do, in fact, see the patients at the bedside with the house staff and students.

Paul R.G. Cunningham, MD, FACS, Dean and Senior Vice Chancellor for Medical Affairs at the Brody School of Medicine at East Carolina University, knew Dr. Stead from North Carolina Medical Society meetings where "I became an admirer of his wisdom and poise":

Clearly everybody in this room is part of the choir. We believe—I believe—that medicine has become so fractionated and so distorted that we think we're practicing a science rather than art form based upon certain scientific principles.

I was a surgeon all of my life before becoming a dean, and Dr. Stead clearly was a surgeon at heart! There's nothing more intimate than teaching *inside* a patient. That is something that is overlooked by all of our students. One of the sentinel points in my teaching is to ask the students when last they did a rectal examination. That requires a level of intimacy that many of them are shy about, which is quite unfortunate. The fact is that we have to be intimate with our patients, and I think Dr. Stead identified that.

R. Sanders ("Sandy") Williams, MD, senior vice chancellor for academic affairs at Duke University, first encountered Dr Stead (and was indelibly imprinted with a number of Steadisms) as a medical student on Long Ward in 1971; thirty years later, while serving as Dean of the Duke University School of Medicine, Sandy again engaged Dr Stead in illuminating conversations about medical education:

Both the articles and the presentations here remind me that the legacy of Dr. Stead is playing out in an important, but curious and unforeseen way—through Duke's new medical school in Singapore. That institution has been established with the primacy of education as its reason to be, and the education there takes place in an environment that's sheltered from the financial and litigation pressures that threaten American medicine. I think many of you would be surprised but pleased to see the extent to which the principles reflected at this symposium are being put in place there. That's no accident because some of the key drivers of the Singapore program, like Frank Starmer, are direct disciples of Dr. Stead. I make rounds there several times a year, and in many ways I feel I have been transported back to 1970 on Long Ward because the environment there is so different from what I see here. The excellence of the physicians dominates, and yes, there's a drive to be fast and efficient in medical care, and a drive to do research of international quality, but education is foremost. I hope that we can use that as a way to promote Dr. Stead's legacy not only across America but worldwide, and to bring some of it back home to Duke.

John Laszlo, MD, a professor at Duke and then Director of the research program at the American Cancer Society, was recruited to Duke by Dr. Stead and Dr. Wayne Rundles; "Stead even gave me a laboratory during my residency, always supported my academic career, and was a great friend and an inspiration for all that I was able to accomplish there":

I want to make one point and ask one question. Very shortly we'll be celebrating the two hundredth anniversary of Charles Darwin and his legacy. I recently heard Professor E. O. Wilson of Harvard, one of the world's great naturalists, comment that theoretical mathematicians reach their peak in their late teens, physicists in their late twenties, molecular biologists in their thirties, and philosophers never. So perhaps this audience is old enough to be in the philosophers' realm. I think we are.

We talk about how time is money, and how we find the patients having all these expensive procedures so they're not in bed on rounds. When Hal Silberman and I were practicing hematology, we did fewer bone marrow aspirations than the trainees because we knew that examination of the peripheral blood often can predict what the bone marrow will show. I've been out of the practice of medicine now for over two decades, but I wonder if a careful history and physical wouldn't substitute ably and at much lesser cost as a trade-off for some of these expensive procedures.

Hal Silberman: I can elucidate for John. I go the lymphoma/leukemia conference every week at Duke, and it's not just the bone marrows that are being repeated. It's two or three PET scans to determine if there's a relapse of a non-Hodgkin lymphoma.

Michael ("Mike") McLeod, MD, a chief resident for Stead and thereafter a clinical gastroenterologist at Duke 35 years, is currently Professor of Medicine, emeritus, and associate director of the Practice Course at Duke University School of Medicine:

One reason the patient needs to be present is to counter our reliance on technology (an abnormal test result) to define disease; if we see the patient, we run the risk that the patient's illness story will not fit the detected abnormality. In gastroenterology we saw patients operated to remove the gall bladder, for instance, and although they had gallstones, their story had nothing to do with the gall bladder. We can't overemphasize the art of a careful history at the bedside, and the importance of hearing the patient's story. The patients are the experts on the story; we're the experts on medicine, and we have to get the two kinds of experts together. When students don't learn the art of history taking, we have all these tests and an excessive reliance on technology rather than understanding what the patient is saying.

Samuel J. Friedberg, MD, Emeritus Professor of Medicine/Endocrinology at the University of Texas Health Science Center at San Antonio, was formerly Associate Professor of Medicine at Duke University Medical Center:

In addition to having been a superb clinician, one of the things that impressed me about Stead was his ability to eliminate artificial roadblocks, the kinds that are pervasive in so many schools of medicine. In the department of medicine at Duke, at least while I was there, there was little internecine fighting; the energy of the faculty was preoccupied with the consequences of his disapproval. He could be brutal at times, but this was how he controlled the behavior of house staff and faculty. You always wanted to please him and remain in his good graces. There was a strong underlying morality and strength of character in the man in his conduct of daily affairs. Although he eschewed the outer trappings and rituals of religion, and was probably an agnostic, in retrospect, I thought his strong religious upbringing was to influence him throughout his life. He was a bit of an ascetic. At the same time, he was not above whatever manipulations were necessary to get things right. In the end, I always felt that whatever he did was not for his own good, but for the good of the department and especially for the good of the of the house staff, and we never felt that we were being used no matter how hard he made us work. Had it not been for him, I would never have achieved the modest success I enjoyed in science. He gave me the opportunity. I often wish he were here to clean up the mess in my present place of employment.

He always terrified me; in his office he would open his desk drawer and fiddle with paper clips, rubber bands, or pencils, and he would then look up at me with deep-set, piercing blue eyes over which hung long bushy eyebrows. What came next, fortunately, was usually a relief. On occasion, my misdeeds came back to me by having been spread through the entire department.

I came away with an understanding of the importance of bedside teaching. In my present position, in another medical school, I made myself unpopular by my insistence on this approach. In fact, I almost had a revolution on my hands, so I explained to the house staff, "You tell me a story about a patient and then, when I see that person, I come away with a completely different impression. You say that this is not a very interesting patient, and when I see the patient, I find him very interesting. You also have to know that the bedside visit is the high point of the patient's day." Now the faculty make rounds in an office, and never see the patient at all. They are too busy treating the computer.

The grand rounds that I attend now are not for the purpose of solving or reviewing a patient's problem. They are not an educational event. They exist for the purpose of showing 60 power-point slides about something or other. I come away having learned nothing. One more point and then I'll shut up. When Gene was eighty-six, he gave a talk at one of Duke's Friday morning conferences. About a month later, he sent me a tape-recording of the event. I had several copies made, and had the effrontery to send them to several higher ups in our school. Nothing rubbed off. I had seen the video a number of times and I was so moved by it that tears welled up, so I showed the tape at our endocrine conference. At the end, all I got was blank stares—they just didn't get it. I guess you just had to have been at Duke at the right time.

Delmer ("Bud") Shelton, PA-C, now retired from Duke and the Durham Veterans Medical Center, came to know Dr. Stead while a Physician Assistant student at Duke; they subsequently became fast friends, visiting each other at their lake homes and often:

It takes a lot of skill to get everyone involved—the teacher must direct comments and questions to learners at different levels, and not everybody is born with those skills. Faculty development programs can help people learn how to do that, how to create an environment in which learners feeling safe as they are learning. There are problems, too, when attending physicians do not feel they have the skills to teach at the bedside, and so it's easier for them not to go there. It is questionable whether learners can learn or teachers can teach when they're scared half to death.

Chapter 3

Learning Is a Community Affair

E. Harvey Estes, MD

A visitor at ward rounds at Duke Hospital in 1945, the year before Dr. Eugene A. Stead became Chairman of the Department of Medicine at Duke, would have found the teaching ward "locked down," with no visitors or unnecessary staff allowed. The beds were all uniformly made up, as if for a military inspection, with the head nurse in full charge of maintaining quiet and order. All nonessential patient care activities were suspended. It would be apparent that this was a special event, led by the Chairman and senior physician, Dr. Frederic M. Hanes. No medical students were allowed and no interns; only residents were permitted. Case presentations were made by a resident physician, followed by a discussion by Dr. Hanes, all in a very formal manner.

This format was so ingrained that when Dr. Stead, upon his arrival, directed Dr. John Hickam to change it to the pattern they had followed at Emory, Hickam seriously questioned whether or not this would be accepted. Dr. Stead insisted, and it was accomplished without major incident. The new pattern was the same as that experienced by all subsequent Stead house officers: all learners joined the faculty member assigned to conduct rounds — medical students, PA students, interns, residents, visiting faculty, nurses, and anyone else who wished to join were packed around the bed. The youngest learner assigned to the chosen patient introduced the patient to the faculty member, and presented the case history, physical findings and lab data. The faculty member would ask questions of the patient, check critical findings, and begin the discussion. The flow of rounds varied with faculty members, but Dr. Stead was likely to drape his frame over the head of the bed and continue the discussion at the bedside. Others would retire to the classroom, much preferred by attendees, since most could sit in a more comfortable setting.

I need not describe these rounds further. Most of you have been there, and done that! The crucial point that I would like to call to your attention is the fact that all learners were there together, and all participated, young and old, neophytes and old hands. In fact, all were learners together. Stead was clearly in charge, but always as a participant, not an autocratic leader (a distinction not always apparent to the junior participants!). The composition and style of the participating group, and the routine and outcome were carefully and deliberately orchestrated for the purpose of training doctors (this was sometimes rendered as training "men," but that descriptor belies the fact that Stead welcomed women from the start).

The Genesis of Stead's Rounding Style

Where did this style of teaching rounds originate? Stead gives credit to Soma Weiss, his mentor at Boston City Hospital:

> Soma had the wisdom to listen to his young staff who described what was known about the disease. He listened to the patient, and asked questions about what was not known about the disease. In the course of the discussion, Soma elected to bring back more information about certain aspects of the problem, and encouraged others to explore areas that had been defined by the discussion. He created a pool of knowledge to which each contributed, and from which each extracted.[1]

Stead's quotation above is a good place to start analyzing the utility and genius of this style of teaching. "He listened to his young staff, who described what was known about the disease." Stead expected each participant to do his or her own research about the problem under discussion. He expected each participant to know the established facts and theories about the illness, and to become familiar with textbooks and the library. Next he "listened to the patient, and asked questions." Stead often commented on Weiss's interest in the presenting complaint of the patient, and collecting information about the ways in which similar complaints could be caused by a wide variety of conditions; Stead continued this legacy. Woe unto the student or resident who brushed away a vague or implausible complaint! The focus was on the patient not the illness, and the family and socioeconomic circumstances in which the patient lived were as important as the disease.

Note, please, that Weiss asked about what was *not* known about the disease. This, too, was a critical feature of Stead's rounds. I recall a case that illustrates this point well. He saw a very obese man on rounds in the mid 1950s, and noted in the course of analyzing the problem that the patient slept a lot, and that his electrocardiogram showed right axis deviation and other features suggesting right ventricular hypertrophy. At that time I was in charge of reading electrocardiograms at the Veterans Administration Hospital. Stead sent the student over with the ECG, asking for a consultation. I had no explanation for the signs of right heart disease, so I wrote my old mentor Dr. Robert Grant, then at the National Heart Institute, asking him whether or not he had encountered such an ECG. He recalled one other case, adding that the findings had reverted to normal when the patient lost weight. This led to discussions and a lot of laboratory research, culminating in a paper by Herb Sieker, Henry McIntosh, George Kelser, and me, describing the pathological physiology of the reversible cardiopulmonary syndrome now known as Pickwickian Syndrome.[2] Sieker was the first person to present the pathophysiology of this syndrome at a national meeting,[3] but others beat us to the draw by publishing the first full paper, and they clearly "aced" us by using the colorful Dickensian name by which it is now known.[4]

Answering Rounds or Questioning Rounds?

In the generation of teachers before Weiss and Stead, rounds emphasized describing disease, making an accurate diagnosis, and providing recommendations for treatment. Stead's predecessor at Emory and Grady Hospital, James E. Paullin was typical of this breed. Paullin was, incidentally, the Stead family physician, and both loved and respected by Stead. His rounds were similar to those of Hanes at Duke in that they were authoritarian rounds, a stage for displaying the knowledge and skills of the senior physician, and dependent on his reputation and experience. Therapeutic choices were few, and the mechanism of action of most treatments was obscure. The experience of the teacher was the basis of his authority, and the information he dispensed was not to be questioned but accepted with the intention that it be absorbed and used as is.

Contrast this to the Weiss/Stead tradition. They expected all learners (including the Chief) to be participants, exploring on their own what was already known about the disease, but then engaging in discussion that sought gaps in knowledge, and questioned current assumptions and conclusions. Questions posed in order to provoke thinking replaced statements to be committed to memory. As often as not, the answers to these questions were not known to Stead or anyone else. The purpose was to stimulate library research, questioning of experts, or going to the physiological laboratory. The result was an ever expanding pool of knowledge, to which all contributed, from which all extracted, and all had fun thinking together. At Stead's rounds, various intellectual positions were clarified and solidified by making a 5-cent wager; the nickel bet was a device that allowed everyone, including the lowest level student, to challenge the "old man" — and to occasionally win!

The composition of the teaching/learning group was important. Students of all levels and types, interns, residents, and faculty were there together. The upper levels had been previously selected by Stead, and were well aware of their role on the team. Stead considered the interaction between the students, interns, and residents to be more important than the faculty-student interaction.[5] The intern and resident had the satisfaction and benefits of teaching, and the student and other junior level learners had the advantage of exposure to teachers that they did not mind quizzing. The function of the faculty was to set the expectations for the outcome and to add to the mix. Everyone was both teacher and learner. No member of the group, junior or senior, was permitted to "opt out" of the discussion. All could be, and were, pulled into the discussion by questions and requests for opinions.

Stead emphasized that there are two effective ways to learn: by doing and by teaching. Little honor was given to mere memorization of facts or regurgitation of received information. Memorized content is quickly lost, and only information that is used and proved useful is permanently imprinted and retained. Because we learn more when we teach than when we are taught, the structure and setting of rounds was designed to allow all to care for patients, and to teach while learning to think and accumulate new knowledge. Stead's rounds were a place in which both doing (caring for patients) and teaching were in full use, for the education of all.

Learning to Doctor

The primary objective of Stead's educational process was to have individuals learn how to care for the sick patient, and how to learn in the complex and ever changing world of medical care. Stead specifically noted that he had no intention of teaching about all diseases, or the best way to treat this disease or that disease. He prodded individuals to approach a patient's problem, ask questions and learn, constantly enlarging their knowledge pool in a way that would last a professional lifetime. He judged the success of the system by the things that happened after the student and teacher parted ways, and by the attitudes and behavior that the students carried into their careers as independent caregivers.

There was no thought of steering a student to a specific specialty, or to a specific activity, such as a career in teaching or research. Stead often noted that his department produced no single product. He recognized the variable ability, proclivities and aims of students, and his objective was to train them all. Many specialists in surgery, obstetrics, psychiatry, and other medical fields benefitted from his teaching. He produced many successful academic leaders, and many superb practitioners of medicine, both generalists and specialists. The point is that the system prepared them all for successful careers.

But we must recognize that the system prepared them to be doctors — professional caregivers who made themselves available to individuals with problems, and who helped their patients in solving their problems. The patient and his or her problem was always the central focus of the process. Research was a means to an end, not an end unto itself. Stead recognized that medical schools and teaching hospitals have an obligation to provide the personnel required to deliver health services to the nation; as early as the mid 1970s he expressed his concern that research was becoming a primary objective of medical education rather than one of an interlocking triad of objectives (along with patient care and teaching).[6] He recognized that this imbalance was a result of the success of research. Research generated financial support, and this brought research-trained physicians, whose career was in the laboratory rather than in patient care, to positions of leadership in medical centers. To quote Stead: "they are producers of new knowledge rather than of men."

He also recognized that the explosive growth in the research leg of the triad was a result of financial investments. The expansion of research facilities, research equipment and personnel was phenomenal, especially when compared to that of teaching facilities and personnel. Adding to the imbalance was the payment system for medical care, which afforded high rewards for technical procedures, low rewards for cognitive services, and no rewards at all for abstract thinking. The question was and still is, can today's medical educational institutions afford the investment of time required for the obviously successful "thinking rounds" of the kind that Stead advocated? This is a question that deserves discussion and debate. How can we alter the reward system to promote the return of balance to the system?

A Synoptic View

Let me summarize my analysis of the Stead legacy in regards to the proposition that *Learning is a Community Affair*. The concept was and is seen at its best in the teaching hospital and in teaching rounds at the bedside. Within this setting, the following components are essential:

1. Learners at all levels of experience are an essential component of the learning process; sharing and interacting contributes to that process. Coaching and preparing those with less experience reinforces knowledge and ensures retention.
2. Emphasis should be placed on what is *not* known, with an expectation that all will seek answers—from reading the literature, from asking experts, and if necessary, from experimental studies. Answers are to be brought back to the group and shared by all.
3. There is no obligation to teach about all diseases, or to gain an encyclopedic knowledge of a specific topic, but there is an obligation to question and to constantly seek information that will plug gaps in knowledge.
4. There are many objectives of this educational process, but the highest priority is given to serving the patient by helping solve the problems imposed by illness. Enlarging the pool of useful, working information available to the student and the group is next. Research is an important way to add to the pool of information, but is a means to that end, and third in rank order. In other settings, such as the research laboratory, this hierarchy of importance might be reversed.
5. Teaching patients about their illness and how to manage it is the ultimate "doctoring" skill.
6. Emphasis should be placed on thinking, not on memorization or displaying an encyclopedic collection of information.

7. Each learner has a unique set of abilities, ambitions, and preferences, which should be recognized and respected. No single combination of learner characteristics is better than another. Everyone benefits from exposure to this teaching environment. All career objectives are respected and served equally.

The Future: Addressing Unknowns

Time and circumstances change all things. As previously mentioned, there is no payment mechanism for support of thinking rounds, so they have largely disappeared from the scene. Today, residents and attending physicians pursue solitary "work rounds," racing to get the day's work done and to satisfy the requirements for payment. Neither students nor the process of producing the practitioners required for care of the population are prime concerns. Procrustean regulations, such as those mandating the maximum length of time that residents can remain in the hospital, make the Stead protocol almost impossible to follow. Can the Stead system be replicated today? We know it works, and most of those who experienced it feel that it is a superior system for educating medical practitioners. Can we achieve the same results with other systems? These are questions we need to discuss.

This symposium documents and describes at least some of the components and processes of Stead's teaching system. We tend to ascribe the impact to Stead himself, but we should remember that he credited Soma Weiss, his chief, with creating the system. It is clear that this teaching method can function and produce results independently of a unique leader. The constraints of the present are largely those imposed by the structure of our reward system, which could be changed by a single act of Congress. As long as we recognize the various advantages of the system, we may be able to preserve the benefits it brings to the patient, to the physician, physician assistant, nurse, and all who will provide care in the future.

In the Steadian tradition of considering what we do not know, I would like to end by proposing some hard realities facing those of us who would like to see Stead's methods and principles incorporated into the medical educational process for future medical professionals. To do this, we must consider how these principles can be transmitted into new settings, such as the community and outpatient settings, which are increasingly important in meeting the needs of both medical teaching and society. How can we provide a base that will include current and new members of the complex medical teams that will be required in the future? How can we use Stead's principles to inspire and recruit primary care doctors, who are increasingly scarce in those areas most in need of care? Finally, how can we insure that the primary emphasis of medical education is responsibility and concern for the patient rather than elucidating the disease process? I hope you will consider these questions, and give us some solutions!

References

1. Stead EA Jr: *A Way of Thinking; A Primer on the Art of Being a Doctor.* BF Haynes, ed. Durham, NC. Carolina Academic Press, 1995, p.64.

2. Estes EH Jr., Sieker HO, McIntosh HD, Kelser GA. Reversible cardiopulmonary syndrome with extreme obesity. Circulation 1957;16:179.

3. Sieker HO, Estes EH Jr., Kelser, GA, McIntosh HD. A cardiopulmonary syndrome associated with extreme obesity (abstract). J Clin Invest 1955;34: 916.

4. Burwell C S, Robin ED, Whaley RJ, Bickelman AG. Extreme obesity associated with alveolar hypoventilation; a Pickwickian syndrome. Am J Med 1956;5:811.

5. Wagner GS, Cebe B, Rozear MP. E. A. Stead, Jr.; *What This Patient Needs is a Doctor.* Durham, NC. Carolina Academic Press, 1978, p.4.

6. Ibid. p.53.

Comments Following "Learning Is a Community Affair"

Ruth Ballweg: I'm impressed by how values are changing in our country today. People talk a lot about "Time." When your kids or your grandkids or your students talk to you, they say, "You're not spending time with me." They don't say, "Give me time"; they talk about "spending," which implies worth and value. It speaks to resources, and I think we need to recognize the amount of time it takes to ensure quality. I agree with Harvey Estes that lack of sufficient quality time is one of the things that patients are angry about. Nobody is giving them the precious resource of their undivided attention.

Bill Stead: I'd like to focus first on new opportunities. We grew up learning from individual patients, and I don't want to stop doing that, but I think we can also learn from a systematic approach to the care of populations of patients. In the past, when a patient was in the hospital for several weeks, we were able to pick up the different aspects of their condition as it evolved. We now have the opportunity to use that kind of longitudinal view to learn systematically how to care for a population; how to translate scientific evidence about a high-risk condition into a standard set of practices that can be appropriately flexed for individual patients; how to develop the roles that will allow people to bring compassion, judgment and wisdom to bear; how to redesign, simplify and standardize process of care; how to use informatics to decrease our dependence on memory and provide a forcing function. How do you actually knit roles, process and technology together to get reproducible results? How can we get our students, who right now are so tied up in scheduled courses that they actually don't have the time to participate in these kinds of activities, to look at these efforts over a period of the three to eighteen months? If they would do so, they would get a new experience that I think might be part of the community approach.

We also have the opportunity to begin to think quite differently about the role of the clinician. I don't know how we want to define that role, but I think we need to keep the person who is going to take responsibility for the patient separate from the technician and from the basic researcher, etc. I think we've got to begin to figure out these fundamentally different roles, which will take fundamentally different approaches to education if we're going to do them well. If we had people with the skills to learn together and to work as a team, while bringing their unique competencies to bear, maybe we could make progress.

Bud Shelton: If you're in a busy practice, seeing fifty patients a day, you'll rarely take as much as twenty minutes, oftentimes less than ten minutes, with a patient or you won't have any time off for sleeping or meals. This is the monster in front of you. And what do the patients see when they enter the exam room? They see the back of a computer. You spend about three minutes talking to the patient and the rest of the time plunking away on this darn keyboard, and then you tell the patient what you put in and what you're going to do, and then greet the next patient. The patient doesn't feel that he's being interacted with because you're spending all your time on the computer. We need to find a way to use the machine but not let it get in the way.

Lois Flaherty, MD, the former head of Child and Adolescent Psychiatry at the University of Maryland, is now retired; she is the Editor of Adolescent Psychiatry:

I graduated from Duke University School of Medicine in 1968; I'm a psychiatrist, a discipline that for a while was a last bastion of doctor-patient interaction, but psychiatry has been affected much the same way as the rest of medicine. That wonderful photo of Dr. Stead at the bedside suggested some ideas to me. We have talked about the intensity of Dr. Stead's gaze but if you look at the photo, it is clear that the patient is a very active participant in the process. That reminds me of one of the very positive things going on in medicine: the consumer movement, which is really very, very strong in psychiatry. I think we need to partner with our patients to change the system. We can't do it ourselves, and patients want change as much as we do. We need to really mobilize them and get together. There's a lot of outrage that hasn't been effectively mobilized to change the whole system—the tort system, the fact that so much of the system of care is controlled by forces presently beyond our control.

The other thing that occurs to me is the importance of developing a team approach to care. This has happened in many areas of psychiatry because we have such a shortage of providers in many parts of the country. We sometimes incorporate medical students or residents, but what we really need is a total team organized according to Dr. Stead's concept of PAs as physician extenders. Maybe we need to really rethink that concept and find ways that people can work together, without having the extenders palpate the abdomen—but not the surgeon. There's got to be a better way of integrating care.

Douglas ("Doug") Zipes, MD, a house officer under Dr. Stead in the 1960s and presently Distinguished Professor at Indiana University School of Medicine, is editor of the journal "Heart Rhythm," co-editor or author of three cardiology textbooks, and author the forthcoming medical thriller, "The Black Widows":

I'd like to pick up on what Bill Stead said because I see a major conflict in how I was brought up—why I went into medicine—and what we have today. Thinking rounds were so much fun because you had the opportunity to be an independent thinker and evaluate the patient and choose a form of therapy. Today "systems" or teams take "care" of patients. You have a set of guidelines that specify what you must do unless you can muster a very good reason for not following them—if you do deviate and the patient subsequently has a problem, you're at risk from a medical legal standpoint.

One medical specialty, anesthesiology, took the systems approach to heart, the way airline pilots use a check-off list prior to takeoff. This reduced anesthesia complications close to zero, and has led to suggestions that cardiology and other areas of medicine do the same thing. Well this seems to me to derail independent thinking because you essentially follow a list of how-to-take-care-of-patients. The electronic medical record is going to have a major impact on this because in many instances the guidelines are built right in. You put in the diagnosis, you get told what to do next. It seems to me there's a conflict between the ability to think for yourself—the fun of medicine—and how to minimize errors.

Bill Stead: These two ideas are not in conflict. A systems approach means that you're trying to do something repetitively *and* correctly, and that is not cookbook medicine. It is in fact systematically looking at the evidence and deciding in a thinking way. Instead of having to do that patient-by-patient, when you think about a population of relatively alike patients, you build thinking into the branch points you to need to use in their care. When you need to vary the protocol, you embed a human in the loop, just like the pilot of a plane who can take over whenever the system seems out of kilter. But when that happens, we need to capture the data so that we can learn whether we do better or worse when the pilot takes over, which allows us to iteratively refine the system. You need to keep in mind that we can have very careful thinking about how to take care of an individual patient; we can have the same kind of thinking about how we take care of a population of patients. We actually want to do both right.

Robin Hunter Buskey, MPAS, PA-C, is with the US Public Health Service; she has held various Physician Assistant leadership positions including membership on the North Carolina Medical Board:

I'm a physician assistant and I want to try to address some of the questions that Dr. Estes posed about community care. I wonder how many in this audience have been following the movement toward group medicine, the provision of services to a group of patients at once, then perhaps bringing individual patients out the group to address individual issues. This could shift how we teach as well as changing the paradigms of community medicine; we might incorporate some of that as we prepare our students for the future.

C. Edward ("Ed") Buckley III, MD, was a medical student, house officer, fellow and young faculty member during Gene Stead's tenure as department chairman; Stead "accepted my suggestion that I practice allergy on the faculty because, at the time, it was the only medical specialty with a creditable focus on and future in clinical immunology":

I'd like to speak to Doug Zipes's point. A number of years ago Max Woodbury and I were looking at probabilities surrounding diagnosis and treatment. We concluded that the assessment of risk that forms the basis of the systems approach is fundamentally flawed and naïve because it does not take into account negative information. Think for a moment about the review of systems. You get a list of positive information and a list of negative information. The mind takes into account that negative information in evaluating the positive information. Somebody with a puffy face and edema could have heart disease; if they have no history of renal disease that probability goes up. Until our systems approach can properly take into account negative information, it's not going to be useful.

Hal Silberman: I took a course on teaching the teacher and it probably was helpful. I'd like to ask how long it takes to teach a teacher to teach. How much does it cost? do some teachers learn faster than others? and, finally, should we tell some would-be teachers that they really shouldn't be teaching on rounds?

Jeff Wong: Well the hours needed vary. One of the enduring myths of medical education is the triple-threat individual who is good at patient care, good at research and good at teaching. In present day academia, we should pay attention to Dr. Estes' notion of separate roles so that the institution comprises a composite triple threat. It would comprise individuals who are very good at research or are excellent clinicians or can teach; it would be a mixture of people. One of my thoughts is that we need to train people who have the inclination or the aptitude to become good teachers, and to support them in a way that allows that to happen. There's a new vogue that started at UC San Francisco and Harvard and Baylor of forming academies of teaching scholars. Ironically, people whose main function in the academic setting is to teach need extra financial support because the time pressure of teaching detracts from seeing patients or obtaining research grants. These academies have sprung up to try to emphasize and support people whose primary role is educating future doctors and learners.

Frank Neelon: Dr. Stead did something remarkable: he put all learners together at the bedside. He did not have separate rounds for beginning students and separate rounds for advanced students and separate rounds for interns and residents. All of these people were at the bedside together, and somehow he was able to get them all learning together. The question is how on earth did he do that? Is that something we can keep doing?

Hal Silberman: Are there individual physicians who really should not be teaching?

Jeff Wong: At the institution where I work, we have people who have become less productive in one way or another and so the thought is, "Then, let them teach." I'm afraid that's happened elsewhere, too. Our present reward system should not encourage people who are not good teachers to continue, but the problem is to find something else for them to do rather than burden learners with people that do not have teaching ability.

Sandy Williams: Doctors, PAs, other caregivers, and patients dislike many elements of the American health system. We've heard from several speakers today how features of that system create obstacles to the type of education, learning and thinking that we'd all like to do. Why is that? The people who run these health systems and hospitals and practice plans are not monsters—in fact, many of them are in this room. I would submit that the people who run governmental programs and insurance companies and pharmaceutical companies are not monsters. They're mostly well-meaning people who are not far off from where we are in their philosophies. So what's the problem? David Lawrence, who used to head the Kaiser system, has spoken eloquently about the problems in the US health care system, and he calls it an impenetrable cocoon of myths, self-interest, greed, habit—lots of things that make it virtually impossible for anyone to take the helm of the health system or a department and change it. There are too many external constraints.

If we learned one thing from Dr. Stead it is that he didn't accept the barriers that tie up other people. That was a dominant feature of his persona. Whatever you said was a reason why something couldn't happen, he would dismiss in a minute, whether it was a patient care issue or something else. So, I'd like to charge everyone — people in this room and others — to do something like that ourselves. We need to find ways around these constraining external forces ways to demonstrate the success of something better. That's what our academic medical centers can do best.

Bill Stead has said many things that are on the right track to a future that will not look like the past. We can't go back to the past. We should never suggest that. The future is going to be something quite different, but it can be quite pleasing in the ways that it's different. I'd like to see academic medical centers band together to get more leverage on the external constraints we have. I hate to be a broken record about this, but I do think there are great opportunities abroad to create new systems and demonstrate that they can deliver better patient care, better education at the same or lower costs than the crazy quilt of American health care or economics.

K. Patrick Ober, MD, Professor of Internal Medicine and Associate Dean for Education at the Wake Forest University School of Medicine, has long admired "the unique Dr. Stead for his exemplary commitment to excellence in patient care, for his great wit, and for his intensely brilliant approach to the education of America's physicians":

As the ambassador from Wake Forest, I am very, very thankful for the opportunity to be here. I've done a lot of background reading about Dr. Stead — an amazingly impressive person. When Dr. Stead went to Emory as chair of medicine, he found he didn't have enough interns or residents to run Grady Hospital because of this thing known as World War II. So he gathered the troops he had (the occasional intern, the occasional resident, medical students, nurses, everybody) and when they made rounds in the morning, they asked each patient, "What can we do for you? what are your expectations?" That's a huge thing we often overlook in our technologically-oriented world: starting off with "What can we do for you?" If we carried on that conversation, I think we would solve a lot of the issues.

The other thing was, he said to the students, "Now is your chance to be a doctor. Because we don't have enough doctors, you can be the doctor. Anybody who wants to opt out can go back to being a student. That's forgivable because you are a student, and we'll let you function at that level. But if you want to up the ante and do something important and meaningful as part of this team approach to patient care, now is the time to do it." If there's any legacy of Eugene Stead's it's to rally the troops together; to be very patient-centered; to break down those barriers that have been getting in our way.

John Laszlo: I'd like to speak to one aspect of Stead's legacy that I think is critical to this discussion, and that was his comfort with saying "I don't know." This is one area where we're not doing a good job training young doctors. When I was responsible for the VA Hospital, we did some experiments with teaching that stemmed from the fact that several second year students couldn't tell me the bases that made up DNA even though they had just finished the course in biochemistry. I thought "Why don't we involve the basic science instructors in teaching rounds on medicine and bring basic science right to the bedside along with the clinical issues." And so I got some of my friends in basic science departments to come on rounds with us. This broke down because you would have biochemists trying to address some neuroscience issue regarding a patient who had a stroke, and they felt totally unprepared. They became very uncomfortable and just couldn't stand being asked questions about what might be going on at the neuron level if that wasn't their area of expertise. Nor do physicians like to be questioned about things they don't know the answers to. We need to do a better job in getting medical students becoming comfortable saying, "I don't know the answer to that but I'll try to find that out."

Mort Bogdonoff: My students carry their Blackberries with them, and when a question comes up to which I don't know the answer, I turn to the MD, PhD student, who pulls out his Blackberry and says, "Well what we need here, Dr. Bogdonoff, is to use this beta blocker as was proven in a study published last week in Circulation." There is complete, immediate access to fundamental science or clinical studies; if you pontificate during rounds, in about five minutes you're proven to be an absolute stupid donkey

because the information about the latest and most effective therapy is readily accessible.

We heard mention of the computer in the doctor's examining
room. Sometimes that screen does sit up there as a distracting men-
ace. It really presents a block because I want to watch what goes in
the room and then type up the history or the physical findings while
the patient is somewhere else. What do you do about recording
data and not have that screen in place?

Bill Stead: Well personally I don't think it's a good use of pa-
tient-physician time for me to ask questions and then type the answers into a computer. It's a much better use of time to help patients
answer certain kinds of questions on their own, with their family,
over the web. That information is then available when we see them,
and we spend our time talking about what it means. I think that we've
got to engage the patient and their support team as a major resource for improving health. Remember my daddy's idea that the
patient is one of the learners, so we actually want to help them answer questions. That doesn't mean that we're abandoning them —
it means we're trying to make them part of the learning team with
us. Then we want to spend our collective time working together;
maybe we will both be looking at a computer screen, but it shouldn't
be just one of us looking at the computer screen.

Chapter 4

We Learn Most When We Ourselves Teach

Earl N. Metz, MD

I was honored to be asked to participate in this tribute to a man who influenced the lives of so many physicians—and physicians' assistants. My perspective is different from that of the other participants. I was never a faculty colleague of Dr. Stead. I spent nine years at Duke, but all in the role of student. I had the good fortune to be assigned to Osler Ward for my first clinical rotation as a junior medical student and again for my first assignment as assistant resident. However, the major impact Dr. Stead had on my career as a doctor and as a teacher came during the year I spent as his chief resident—I believe I was the next to last of his residents. He was always kind to me and to my wife but, even after many years, I remained so in awe of him that I never called him Gene. He was always Dr. Stead to me and to my family.

If we are to talk about teaching as a way of learning, there may be no way to improve on the lessons I learned at the bedsides on Osler Ward at Duke during Dr. Stead's time as Chairman.

Dr. Stead thought outside the box before that concept became a cliché and an expression used to describe anything resembling original thinking no matter how trivial the subject. Every student or resident who spent time with Dr. Stead came to expect that he would come up with something in the patient's history or the physical examination that we had overlooked, but which ended up being the deciding factor in the diagnosis or the disposition. I always wondered how he did it. Could he read minds? Did he have access to information we didn't know about? Was he a genius? I realized years later that he was indeed a genius, but a gentle genius who cared, who could make the most humble tobacco farmer in North Carolina believe that he was the most important patient in Duke Hospital. We didn't understand exactly how he did this and were perhaps a bit envious. Dr. Stead could spend twenty minutes with our patient and was, from then on, the one of us the patient remembered. I recall especially a patient who was admitted to Osler Ward late in the evening, who turned out to have an acute surgical abdomen, and was about to be transferred emergently to the surgical service. When I presented our plan to the patient he said, "Son, nobody operates on me unless Dr. Stead says 'OK.'" I called Dr. Stead and told him about our problem. Dr. Stead told me to tell the patient that he said to go ahead with the surgery then said, "Tell him 'Hey' for me."

After nine years at Duke and two years in the military, my family and I returned to Ohio where I spent the next thirty years practicing medicine and teaching at the Ohio State University Medical Center. It was the right move for us but I often wondered, especially during my early years at Ohio State, if the Stead influence was too obvious. We all want to create our own identity but it's difficult to spend time under the influence of a master and not come away concerned about the comparison. I had been recruited to Ohio State by Dr. James Warren, and spent the next twenty years working with him. Dr. Warren had been a colleague of Stead's in Boston, at Emory, and at Duke. Jim was also an exceptional medical scholar who, like Dr. Stead, had a way of putting complicated topics into clear perspective. He helped me understand my hero. He said that if you gathered together the one hundred best internists in the country and presented them all with the same clinical question, ninety-nine of them would come up with a similar answer. Dr. Stead would be one hundred eighty degrees off from the others but, if you gave him twenty minutes, the other ninety-nine would be convinced that he was correct. That's the Dr. Stead I knew on Osler Ward.

Learning from Informal Teaching

Teaching and learning are so closely related that it's difficult to separate them. During my medical student days with Dr. Stead, it never crossed my mind that he might be learning while he taught us. Later, when he sent us off to consult about difficult problems with faculty members in other divisions or departments, I began to understand that perhaps both the teacher and the student were going to benefit. Dr. Stead had a mind that was so different from what most of us have that there is nothing to be gained by comparison or by envy. On the other hand, there is much to be gained by using the insights that came from his genius to improve our own teaching and patient care. A teacher cannot be effective if the problem at hand cannot be expressed in simple terms that can be understood by a first year medical student or, more importantly, by the patient.

My assigned topic today suggested that I first concentrate on the role of a physician as a teacher of medical residents and medical students. There is no doubt that a teacher of medical students must understand pathological anatomy, pathophysiology, and appropriate therapeutics well enough to make it all clear to a student who has not faced the problem before. In fact, true genius in teaching is the ability to put complex principles into simple language that is understandable to both colleagues and patients. Anyone who has spent much time as a teacher knows that nothing makes a concept as indelible as trying to make it clear to someone who has never thought about it before. For me, the physical examination is the best example. Since my Osler Ward days, the fine points of the physical examination have been the most satisfying part of bedside teaching. I made teaching rounds at Ohio State daily for six to nine months a year for almost thirty years. I became pretty good at the physical examination—by pointing out to students and residents what could be learned from examining the finger nails, listening over blood vessels in different positions, using the soft percussion technique I learned from Dr. Cooper on the TB Ward at the Durham VA Hospital, looking into the eye grounds with the patient sitting, even using the electric motor on the bed to raise it up to waist level to make the examination more comfortable for both patient and physician, and, finally, examining with a gentle touch. It's difficult to feel the liver or spleen or axillary lymph nodes if the hand and extended fingers are used like a spear. Teaching and learning medicine is a complicated interaction among trainees, physicians, and patients. The more I taught physical examination, the better examiner I became. The proof always came from patients who said, "No one ever examined me like that before."

Everyone who teaches has a favorite example of teaching the simple facts of pathophysiology in a way that gets the point across. In my specialty, hematology, it has always been frustrating to be called to see a post-operative patient with polycythemia whose high hemoglobin value had been thought to be an advantage going into the operating room. It's been known for years that the surgical morbidity of operating on patients with untreated polycythemia is in the range of seventy percent. That excess morbidity is brought to normal simply by removing enough blood to produce a normal hemoglobin value before the surgery. I've read several explanations for the excessive surgical bleeding in patients with polycythemia, but none makes the problem as clear as my own simple-minded explanation that occurred to me when I was eating an overly ripe peach. I got peach juice all over me. Patients with a much expanded blood volume are like a ripe peach — every available capillary is filled with blood. When you have a chance, compare eating a crisp apple to a ripe peach. I've always searched for simple analogies to explain complex pathophysiology — especially when the precise pathophysiology is not clear. I remember a similar analogy used to describe right ventricular hypertrophy in patients with mitral stenosis. It might have come from Dr. Harvey Estes — at least I've always given him credit for it. The analogy is that filling the left ventricle in a patient with mitral stenosis is like trying to blow up a truck tire using a Penrose drain between the pump and the tire. No wonder the right ventricle gets overworked. There must be many, many more. I wish I knew them all so I could have taught them.

The Value of Skilled Examination

Unfortunately, both the physical examination and the medical history have become, for many, a perfunctory exercise to be completed like grace before a meal—so we can get on with the "real business" of medicine. What a shame! Some of our brightest young academicians seem to be searching for ways to make real patients obsolete in medical training. Trained actors have become standard subjects for medical students learning how to take a history. I suppose there's nothing fundamentally wrong with that concept but why, when there are so many live patients out there hoping to see a live physician, can't we bring them together to meet with live medical students who will share their common goals? The same problems are magnified in teaching the physical examination. We now have plastic dummies constructed to simulate most of the important parts of human anatomy. Again, I suppose that's not a terrible way to train medical students. For example, if it's possible to construct an accurate model of the human oropharynx of approximately the appropriate plasticity, and to use the model to teach the technique of endotracheal intubation, I'd think that would be an appropriate first step before trying it on a desperate patient. On the other hand, I can't think of any compelling reason why the major portions of the physical exam should be learned in any way but on the real thing. The plastic dummies can't say "Ouch!" when the examiner is too rough.

I write what follows without a hint as to whether or not Dr. Stead would agree or would come up instead with one of his 180 degree alternatives. What I have learned, and believe firmly after years of medical practice and teaching medicine, is that patients know the difference between a smart young doctor and a doctor, young or old, who really cares—the way Dr. Stead did for years on Osler Ward. It took several years for me to put the teaching-learning relationship into a clear focus, but time and age have clarified things a bit. First of all, learning medicine in the company of a master clinician, even a master like Dr. Stead, is not a one way street. What made "teaching rounds" on Osler Ward so special was that the patient, the medical students, the house staff, and Dr. Stead were all equal participants and equal beneficiaries; if anyone was given an advantage, it was the patient. Perhaps the most important aspect of the learner as teacher concept is learning to pass on to the patient what is known and what is unknown about the situation, and doing it in a way that makes it clear that a caring physician will be available — whatever comes to pass.

Learning from More Formal Teaching

Perhaps the most satisfying teaching for a physician comes from those special situations that involve a patient, a group of young physicians, and a real bedside dilemma. On the other hand, the most precise teaching-learning experience comes with formal classroom teaching when a topic must be presented to a group of peers. The material may consist of data derived from your own research or from your interpretation of the work of others but in either case the presentation must be prepared with precision and critical interpretation so that it will withstand the critical judgment of experienced peers. Well prepared formal presentations probably leave as indelible an imprint on the brain of the presenter as does a stroke of genius at the bedside.

If bedside teaching and classroom lectures are great learning experiences for the teacher, then writing for peer review may be the ultimate teacher-learner experience. All of us who have dealt with editorial boards know that being less than completely sure of your facts leads to a frustrating outcome. But either positive or negative outcomes with editors can lead to genuine learning — often to new ways of thinking about the material you submitted. Not every clinician has accepted the challenge of writing for peer review, but there is perhaps nothing as clarifying for the intellectual soul as presenting your thoughts to a critical editor.

The New Environment of Education

We need to take some time to consider what the lessons learned on Osler Ward have to do with the study of medicine today—and whether or not they are even relevant. To begin, the exchange of money for the provision of medical care has changed so much in the past fifty years that it has become the driving force for nearly every aspect of what we do. Fifty years ago, Duke Hospital charged a flat rate of twenty six dollars a day for inpatients and the twenty six dollars covered just about everything. Today we charge that much for a single tablet of acetaminophen. When I joined the house staff at Duke, interns were paid twenty five dollars a month. The interns who just started at my university hospital will be paid almost forty five thousand dollars a year; the sad thing is that, as much as that may seem to be, it's not enough to pay the cost of malpractice insurance for some of our colleagues. The yearly premium for my first malpractice policy was thirty-two dollars. What has become obvious is that a lot of money is changing hands for medical care. Doctors are still paid well but, to receive their share, they have been forced to practice in ways that would not be recognizable to our patients on Osler Ward in the 1950s and 60s. Leisurely bedside rounds have become an unaffordable luxury. Yet there is no way to improve on the three essentials of medical care derived from bedside rounds whether in the hospital or in an outpatient clinic: teaching, learning, and care of the patient all converge in a mutually beneficial way that can't be duplicated by any of the contrived devices designed to accomplish these outcomes in isolation from one another.

What I learned from Dr. Stead on Osler Ward, and what has been confirmed many times over during thirty years of making bedside rounds at Ohio State, is that the student, the house officer, the attending physician, and especially the patient all have their own special knowledge about the situation that the others don't have. The best medical decisions result from pooling that information. Isn't it a shame that, to save precious time today, what passes for the medical history may be written up from old records before the patient even arrives at the hospital! If such a history were presented to Dr. Stead, it would take him about a minute to turn his attention away from the presenter and to the patient.

And if the medical history has been condensed and abridged to the point that the patient wouldn't recognize it, the physical examination has suffered even more. Dr. Stead carried his own ophthalmoscope and was better at using it than any of us—in fact, he is holding it at the bedside of a patient in my favorite photograph of him. I discovered a couple of years ago that none of our medical residents carries an ophthalmoscope. The problem is perhaps even worse when it comes to the cardiac examination. Between lessons from Dr. Stead and Dr. Harvey Estes, I became at least passable at listening to the heart. My hope was that the advent of echocardiography would make auscultation of the heart even more accurate and precise. Quite the opposite has happened. The physical examination of the heart is now recorded in the most non-committal terms possible so that an echocardiogram can be ordered (and then it is reported in equally non-committal terms). The results of a carefully performed physical exam should be the basis for interpretation of the technical studies that follow. It should be fun for the examiner and at least interesting for the patient.

Clinical Learning Is Uniquely Cooperative

Among the scientific disciplines, medicine is unique in that the teacher, the student, and the subject are all living, thinking beings, capable of contributing to the knowledge pool that leads to appropriate decision making. I'm convinced that there is no better way to transfer and expand medical knowledge than to make it a group effort with a living patient at the center of the group. The result of that interaction should come out in favor of the patient.

How then are we to teach and learn medicine in a way that advances the science and the art? It can't happen if physicians are so busy trying to meet requirements for "documentation" that patients and students are pushed into the background. It can't happen if we try to teach physical examination techniques using plastic dummies while thousands of living patients want to see a living doctor.

Dr. Stead had it right. There is no better way to learn or to practice medicine than to bring together the interested parties with the patient as an equal and respected partner. The fact that this has become increasingly difficult to accomplish doesn't mean it should be abandoned. What we must do to provide the best medical education and optimum patient care is to reorient and redesign the system in such a way that the care of the sick and the education of medical students and house staff are all served in a way pioneered by William Osler and refined, perhaps even improved, by Dr. Stead on Osler Ward at Duke.

It has now been almost fifty years since my experiences with Dr. Stead began. I can relive some of those moments as though they happened last week. That sharp recall of remote events may simply be a part of the aging process, but I hope that I'm not alone with those feelings, and that others from other places and other times may help exert pressure to bring both the learning and practice of medicine back to where it belongs—to the patient. If the Osler-Stead approach to learning, teaching, and practicing medicine is best for all concerned, then there is no argument in favor of letting business concerns drive us to settle for anything less than the best.

Comments Following "We Learn Most When We Ourselves Teach"

Earl N. Metz, MD, is a graduate of the Duke School of Medicine, a product of the residency in internal medicine and fellowship in hematology at Duke, and a disciple of Dr. Stead's for fifty years:

This has been a really interesting morning to me, and I have changed what I was going to say two or three times as I sat here. I kept thinking of those wonderful old beer commercials featuring Boog Powell and a nearsighted umpire. At the end, the umpire said, with a wonderful southern accent, "I still don't know why they asked me to be in this commercial." The only thing that qualifies me to be here is that I spent thirty years making bedside rounds, six or usually seven days a week, for most months of the year. And even though I've been asked to talk about how you integrate teaching and learning that seems to me to be so obvious that it really does not need much discussion.

I am strongly biased toward the proposition that the only way to teach and learn medicine is in the presence of a patient. That's the only way the learning sticks. There are lots of ways to augment short-term memory from a textbook, but the only way to make the information stick is by a field trip to the bedside of a patient accompanied by other people who are interested in learning some medicine. Dr. Stead did that beautifully. His mind, of course, was one in a million, and to make it even more interesting, he knew that. He knew how his mind worked and how to bring that knowledge to bear on the patient and on us. He knew how to teach medicine.

One irony of this symposium is that we're talking about the teaching legacy of Dr. Stead, and he would be the first to disclaim that he taught anything. "I'm not your teacher. I don't know how to teach. Only you can learn. I can't teach you anything." And yet he was the master-teacher at the bedside. We probably ought to say again and again and again that that wonderful picture of him looking at that patient really says it all. In the brief notes that precede these comments, you'll see a vignette about Dr. Stead with a patient who was admitted to Osler Ward but urgently needed to go to the operating room. He said, "Son nobody operates on me unless Dr. Stead says it okay." That was the result of a previous admission where Dr. Stead spent twenty minutes at the bedside and made that kind of lasting impression. He could make anybody in Duke Hospital feel as though they were the most important person in that hospital, and it stuck.

My beginnings at Duke were inauspicious. My first clinical rotation as a Duke medical student was on Osler Ward in September of 1959. The first night I had to work up a patient to present to Dr. Stead the next morning, so I stayed up all night until finally taking a break at about 6:00 AM. Dr. Stead came to rounds and of course I was terrified. I did my best with the patient presentation I had worked on all night, and when I was finished he looked at all of us around the bedside and said, "Does anyone have any idea what's going on with this patient?" I thought it was all over. I had given it everything I had and failed totally and I was never going to be a doctor—and that's the kind of relationship I had with Dr. Stead all the years. Even when he asked me to be chief resident he said "You know we have a lot of people on this house staff who would be good chief residents, but I think this job would do you some good."

How can you turn that down? I took the offer and it was more than worthwhile. I don't want to be too cute about this because what Dr. Stead did is in a way easy. It's very easy. All you have to do is go to the bedside with a genuine curiosity—which he always had—and be interested in the patient, and transmit your care and your interest in the Francis Weld Peabody sense. Teaching and learning come from that. And when you care and are interested, you make the best medical decisions. You just have to be confident in what you're doing, and be comfortable with what you don't know, and that's the essence of his rounds. He approached things in the sense of "Isn't that interesting. I don't really understand this, but what can we do to figure it out?" And as students and residents working with him, we would go off to see this chief and that surgeon, and come back and report to him. And that's how we learned.

I am concerned that we don't do that very much anymore. People like Dr. Bogdonoff are the last hold-outs for bedside rounds. It's a shame. It's a shame that not everybody does it because that's where the patient is, that's where learning takes place, and patients appreciate it. I have never been sued for making bedside rounds. I've never had a patient say don't bring that bunch around here again. It's enjoyable. It's fun. It's the best part of medicine and we are at fault for letting that fall through the cracks.

Much money changes hands these days, but we have to find a way to direct more effort toward what we are talking about here because that's what patients care about. We can't spend two million dollars a year on a hospital administrator's salary or ten million on the administrator of a health care insurance plan. Doctors make out just fine. We are not underpaid, although I know some generalist internists who are scraping by. But we have to make sure that medicine directs money toward what really counts—taking care of sick people. What really puts medicine into perspective for me is something we never talk about—the fact that every one of those patients is going to die. Some will die before we do. Some will die after we do. But they're all going to die, yet we behave as though, if we do everything right, that's not going to happen. But it is, and when the time comes for me, I hope that there is a tall, gangly, slow-talking Georgian who comes in and hangs on the bed frame and says, "Well now, what can I do for you."

Ruth Ballweg: I really think the key issue is curiosity. Medical schools talk about "problem-solving." Well, problem solving is very goal oriented. It sounds like all you need is an algorithm, and there's no need for a person in the process. When I think about the best teachers, and when I hear stories about Eugene Stead and people trained by him, there's this open-ended curiosity that really pervades the point of view. We all want to have our students develop that over time, and that seems like the central theme.

Bill Stead: There's one piece of my father's legacy that might be important here, but hasn't been mentioned. He and Mother always lived below their income. They entertained students and faculty at the same level that the students and junior faculty could afford to entertain others. My father felt that you should be paid less for thinking because it was enjoyable, and you should be paid more for running in a rat race. As I listen to the tone of this discussion, I wonder whether our profession has abdicated some of these values.

The way we care for individual patients "in the system" usually makes no sense when we really look at it. Therefore the opportunity to improve it is huge. It's not ten percent, it's forty to sixty percent. There's a huge opportunity available if we want to figure out how to do things right; we could free up time and money to be redirected to solving the problems we want to solve. Maybe it is as simple as beginning to get people to take responsibility for the patient, and unwind the spiral.

Jeff Wong: Earl Metz has emphasized how important it is that teachers have a relationship with learners. That is the reason that you were so taken with Dr. Stead—he was very interested in you, in your growth as an individual. Teachers need to make their learners feel that they are taking care of the most important patient in the hospital. That's not easy. There are people in academia now who don't feel the need for that relationship with learners. I don't know if can be instilled, but it may be a key element that's missing. We don't have enough teachers with a vested interested in making sure that every one of their learners actually improves. They're busy with what they're doing, and lose sight of what being a mentor means.

Charles ("Chuck") Hayes, MD, first encountered Dr. Stead during his junior medicine clerkship on Osler Ward; he was later asked by Ike Robinson to develop a hemodialysis program. Dr. Stead allowed just one RN for the program, so "we trained former military corpsmen as dialysis technicians, and several of them entered the first class of Stead's famous PA program":

I'm from Jacksonville, Florida, and was at Duke for a number of years in the 1960s. Most people here seem to think it would be a great idea to go back to teaching at the bedside and fostering a closer interaction of faculty and students, but fret about how to do that in the present environment. We need to remember that the environment was not very good when Dr. Stead came to Duke. The problems were different, but there were problems. And Dr. Stead virtually dropped everything else to put his full attention on this particular problem. He rounded on Osler Ward 11 months out of the year. He quit doing research—he went around and checked up on everybody else doing research, but his job was running the teaching program, and he did it magnificently even though in the early years it was pretty difficult. There were problems getting going, but by the time I came along Stead's way was the accepted way. I think that someone's going to have to take over a program and commit their life to getting this teaching job done.

John B. ("Jack") Emery, Jr., MD, FACP, former chief of medicine at Permanente Medical Group in both Portland, OR and Raleigh, NC, is currently a part-time internist at Rex Senior Center in Raleigh; as a Duke student in 1963, he had his senior exam from Dr. Stead, but never rounded with him:

My observations concern the changing attitudes of young physicians as they come through the educational system, and how we have to manage them after their training. We've talked a great deal about what a wonderful time our gray and balding heads had, but what I see from the professorial perspective troubles me: the changing attitudes of the incoming students, their demands — not their technological proficiencies, but their expectations of what they're going to get out of medicine, and what's going to be the quid-pro-quo for them. Their attitudes trouble me. We may feel wonderful because we've been there, we sacrificed, we learned, but somehow attitudes have shifted, and I wonder what was once so wonderful can even be relevant today.

Again I'm old, but I see a diminished work ethic, an increased demand by young doctors for what the system can give them, and very definite ideas about how much work they're willing to put forth. I don't mean this as a put-down on younger people, but I've been watching this shift in attitude for 27 years, so this is not an instantaneous observation. And I'm curious about their attitude toward the teaching process. We've heard about it only from our side, not from their side.

Andrew G. ("Andy") Wallace, MD, a medical student, house officer, chief resident, and faculty member at Duke under Dr. Stead, was later chief of cardiology and CEO of the hospital at Duke, and then dean at Dartmouth Medical School:

I left Duke in 1990 to become the Dean of the Medical School at Dartmouth for 10 years. A grocer who was one of my former patients gave me some money so that I could have lunch with students every week throughout the year. I'd like to respond to Dr. Emery's question by giving my impressions based on Dartmouth and other schools that I visited. Not all, but most students enter medical school with a set of laudable values about what they want to achieve in life, and what they want to do. They espouse a willingness to work, and the right ethic about the matters we are discussing today. But something happens as they traverse medical school (and even more, their residencies) that produces the signs and symptoms that Dr. Emery describes. Part of this has to do with the fact that the system in which they are being taught does not lead to the kind of ethos and ethic we say we want, even though it may produce terrific technical skills and so on. I like to believe that our students have the raw material and the right attitudes but that something happens to them.

Harvey Cohen: It's pretty clear that the generation that's now coming into medicine, both medical students and those a little older, has values very different from ours. They tend to see medicine as a business, and they have a different level of expectation about family life, about personal life, about their free time compared to what they do in medicine. This has a marked influence on how people view both their training and their ultimate careers. I don't say that as condemnation; it's simply the way it is, and I think we will do ourselves a disservice if we ignore that or don't try to accommodate to it in our approaches to training.

I just want to ask one question to get people to think a little bit more about Harvey Estes's talk and what Earl Metz said. Increasingly in internal medicine, we hear about the push towards the outpatient arena in both practice and in training. We've talked a lot about the joys of bedside teaching but mostly in the inpatient arena. And I'd like to ask how (and I'm not sure we can), how we can bring Dr. Stead's principles of teaching and learning to the outpatient arena. That is increasingly the place most people see as necessary for training. I'm not taking that as given, but we need to address that.

Stuart Bondurant, MD, a house officer and Fellow (with John Hickam) in the Department of Medicine at Duke, subsequently had a career in academic medicine similar to that of Gene Stead, of which in 1974 he said, "It's been a great adventure":

I now live in Chapel Hill, but my roots are at Duke from way back. I want to comment on the exchange between Andy Wallace and Harvey Cohen. I must have done something very bad in a prior life because I've now been dean of three medical schools, and I comment from that perspective regarding the current generation and its values. I really think that both Andy and Harvey are correct. I agree with Andy that they come in relatively unexposed to what we see as negative values, but they quickly reach the point that Harvey described. That is a problem, but Harvey's broader point is the one that's really important: these students reflect a broad social and cultural change. In most of the discussion that's gone on today about the doctor-patient relationship, about how we communicate to patients, we've really not mentioned once, for example, text messaging. Text messaging is now the most conventional way of communicating short term, but I just pick that as one example of the extent to which technology has changed the culture. It seems to me that one of Stead's great legacies was his ability to look at the world as it really is. He had a clarity of definition that really was quite exceptional. We need to look with Steadian eyes at the world as it really is, and as it's going to be, and that will cause us to change some of our directions. I particularly liked Bill Stead's idea we can bridge the gap between population medicine and individual medicine to the mutual benefit of both.

I think that the expectations of our patients are going to be different in the world to come compared to what they were in the world that's past. The healthcare system is going to change, perhaps violently, over the next 20 or 30 years. That makes it especially important that some of the fundamental considerations that have been on the table today, and the marvelous papers that have been read, will serve as a source of influence when the system does change.

Doug Zipes: I'm fortunate never to have been a dean, but I have been a Chief of Cardiology, and speaking from that perspective, I absolutely agree with what Harvey Cohen said. Young doctors today, particularly those from American medical schools, apply for cardiology fellowship and ask questions that, had I asked them of Dr. Stead, would have gotten me fired before I was hired. They are overwhelmingly interested in "quality of life," in hours on duty, in how much they will be paid, and so on. The young people who are "eating their lunch" come from the Middle East and the Far East. *These* kids want to work 12 or 16 hours a day as most of us did in our training. *They* are getting the fellowships, the research opportunities, and so on. I'm the editor of a heart journal, and some years ago I asked Dr. Stead to write an article on making rounds, having been as impressed as all of us were with rounds at Duke.

He said, "I'm not making rounds anymore." When I asked why, he said, "Because the students and house staff are no longer interested in the questions that I ask." I found that a very, very sad commentary, but a testimony to the new crop of youngsters today.

One last point: We've heard much about what Dr. Stead contributed, but I was struck by Joe Greenfield's paper because one of the things that Dr. Stead did was to scare the hell out of us. We've heard anecdotes about how all of us were frightened by him, but we're here today to revere him. What was it that he was capable of doing? You could hear our sphincters snap shut when he walked on to Osler ward, yet we're all here to dedicate this day to his memory. One of the things that did strike me was his incredible ego strength so that he was not afraid to be wrong. And that gives you an incredible amount of freedom to be right.

Elizabeth Ross, DPT, MMSc, a faculty member in the Division of Doctor of Physical Therapy in the School of Medicine, is connected to Eugene Stead by this symposium and the reflections of others:

I teach physical therapy at Duke and in the Practice Course where beginning medical students are introduced to clinical thinking, so I can comment on students today. I do think that, when they come, they share the same values as most of us in this room, but they also take their cues from us. The connections we make with them are very powerful and very important to them. And teaching is connection. Connections made in the first year have to be carried through when they go out onto the wards, otherwise the classroom connection doesn't seem real to them. That's one of the big problems.

I also think that there's less focus today on the role of physician as teacher. I don't think medical students get enough education about education, which is important because they will be teaching their patients. Understanding how they learn and how their patients learn would be valuable for them. They may be getting introduced to a culture of medicine that is changing, but it's up to us to help them understand how to hold on to their values. Connection is what is important.

Mort Bogdonoff: It is my impression that the students now entering medical school are actually better scholars and more talented in many different ways than we were. One of the reasons is the number of women who have joined the profession. Look around this room: the former chief residents are all men. Well, at Cornell over the past 10 years, many of the Chief Residents have been women, a consequence of having doubled the pool of candidates without increasing the number of students going to medical school. As a result, we've raised the level of the talent and also changed who we are. Women in medicine have brought entirely different work demands regarding their lives in the profession. That has to be taken into account when you demand that 16 hour days are necessary.

Earl Metz: I agree with Andy's assessment of how things have changed, and how the students change during the course of medical education. My bias is that the change has occurred because fewer and fewer faculty physicians bear any measure of Dr. Stead's characteristics. Over the past 20 years, the size of our hospital has increased four-fold with a relatively small increase in the number of beds. Still, the house staff is at least twice as big as it was 20 years ago, and the number of faculty is ten times larger. And no one has any time. We've got all these people, and they say they just don't have time to go see the patient. I don't understand it. What are they doing all day?

Hal Silberman: I want to come back to Dr. Metz's point about teaching. I don't know whether he still believes in "see one, do one, teach one," but how does this apply, say, to a procedure? How does it apply to a resident who's going to teach a student do an LP? How many LPs on live patients are required to be good in practice?

Earl Metz: I think the question of how many you have to do to be qualified is being taken out of our hands by regulations at the national and hospital level. For certain procedures, practice on models and dummies may help (it's safer to practice a hundred times on the dummy before you try to intubate your first patient who desperately needs an endotracheal tube). With regard to being smart and being a doctor, my comment has always been that you don't have to be a genius to be a good doctor, although that's not a handicap.

E. Harvey Estes, MD, a resident under Stead in 1952–53 and thereafter a faculty member in his department, became chair of Duke's new Department of Community and Family Medicine in 1966 (with continuing responsibility for Stead's new Physician Assistant program); he retired in 1990 as Emeritus Professor of Community and Family Medicine:

I want to go back to Bill Stead's suggestion that we might solve some of these problems by making a corporate entity responsible for the many things that the individual doctor once did. I think the comment about embedding a human in the loop is absolutely on the mark. In many offices, the human in the loop is the telephone operator. If the patient gets a telephone operator who is responsible, and can find a person to answer the patient's question, that's sufficient. A corporate entity that embeds warm humans who can talk to other humans and make them feel that they are being listened to, who is responsible for passing on the patient's complaint or request or whatever, that's adequate. It can be done and it can be done easily.

Bill also mentioned that the patient has got to be a part of the loop. Patients in general are pretty smart people, particularly about the things that bother them. Sometimes they know more than we know. I'm interested in how we can harness that knowledge by getting patients to talk to one another and perhaps be their own caregiver in many circumstances. Gene Stead said that 80% of what adult patients bring into the office has no cure. Think about that. Like the osteoarthritic problems that are rampant among us, 80% of what adult people bring into the doctor's office cannot be cured. The only answer is to teach the patient to take care of himself, and to get in touch with us if something comes up that we might help. Patients have to learn to manage themselves, for the most part. I think we are a little bit arrogant to think that we can cure even a small percentage of the people who walk in our door. Our ultimate job is to teach patients how to handle themselves and their own illnesses, and Gene Stead said that many, many times. Your job is to teach the patient to be his own doctor. Any successful healthcare plan of the future will have to make the patient a very active part of the system. In many cases, they are more determined to find answers than their physician is, and they can afford to spend a lot more time at it. They are the unknown asset that we have to harness for the future; we should weave them into any healthcare solutions we come up with.

Joseph C. ("Joe") Greenfield, Jr., MD, is a cardiologist who served as the Chairman of the Department of Medicine from 1983–1995; he considers "Dr. Stead to be my primary role model both as a physician and leader":

I want to comment on what Andy Wallace said because I think, in large measure, he's quite right. I'm not even sure when the menu changed for the people coming in, but the menu has certainly changed, and what we do to them is not good. I think that probably this is best highlighted by a 1987 study done by one of our chief residents who gave beepers to house staff on call. The beepers sounded randomly, at which time the house officers wrote down what they were doing. We repeated the study seven or eight years later, and the difference was perfectly obvious: in 1987 the junior residents and the interns spent 50% of their time in the presence of the patient, carrying out activities directly related to patient care; now it's dropped to 25%. I still attend on the Coronary Care Unit, and inevitably, when I walk on to the Unit, the house staff is sitting around that damn computer, looking at it. What is basically a servant that should be under our control is now running the show. They worry a lot more about what's on the computer than what's going on with the patient. And that's not a trivial problem.

The other problematical thing we've done is to tell students that they've just got to sleep all night long, that they shouldn't stay up because it's bad for them, and they shouldn't be in the hospital, and all that. As far as I'm concerned, that's just total, unmitigated nonsense. We have gotten ourselves into this situation because we've made the house staff so big because we have to have so many damn people covering because they can't work. It's a serious problem, and I have no idea why we've allowed it to happen, but I think we have moved the focus from the patient to the computer. Now the house staff has got to spend at least two-thirds of their time in the hospital figuring out how to get out of the hospital. So it's not a simple problem.

Paul R. G. Cunningham: I clearly sense the strong anxiety of almost everyone in the room that we not lose the humanity that Dr. Stead so ably transmitted. He had, it appears, a personal naiveté coupled with a very hard side that he managed very, very well. Nobody would take him for a fool, nor would he put up with nonsense. What I saw in the face of that African American patient looking up at Dr. Stead was a plea for hope; perhaps that's one of the things that we, as physicians, need to learn how to provide. Many of the diseases that we attempt to treat, even in our modern world of CT scanners, computers, PET scanners and other technological advances remain incurable. We can still feel good in that we can provide hope.

Chapter 5

Thinking Trumps Memorization: The Lesson on Attending Rounds?

Joseph C. Greenfield, Jr., MD

The primary title of this presentation, "Thinking Trumps Memorization," implies that the higher level of cerebral function (thinking) is of significantly greater importance. As with any discussion, it is essential to first define, as precisely as possible, what one is talking about. The American Heritage Dictionary provides the following definition of the word thinking: "a way of reasoning; judgment."[1] The same dictionary defines the word memorize as: "commit to memory; learn by heart." The issue in question is the degree to which each of these interrelated functions is essential in the development of the clinical judgment needed by a competent physician. Clearly, if we were to quantify the percentage of each factor needed by a theoretical physicist, thinking would be dominant. However, opera stars such as Luciano Pavarotti or Enrico Caruso would have found it impossible to "think" their way through an operatic aria unless they had committed the words to memory.

Information: Storing It

Dr. Stead describes the relative importance of the two cerebral functions in a paper entitled "Thinking Ward Rounds."[2] He takes the position that if one spends too much time memorizing, there will be little time to think. Obviously, he rates thinking as of paramount importance. On the other hand, he admits that without adequate bits of knowledge, there would be no thinking. That's the rub. The issue is the definition of adequate. Perhaps it might be informative to consider the role of memory, as opposed to thinking, in physicians whom we consider outstanding. In my opinion, most of these doctors have heads crammed with facts—they rely primarily on memory. Dr. Stead's contemporary, the internationally acclaimed Dr. Jack Meyers, and Dr. Ralph Corey, a master clinician at Duke University Medical Center (DUMC), are excellent examples. Although they clearly use thinking to organize their facts, without a vast knowledge base, they would not have been able to function at the highest level as physicians. In comparing the relative importance of these cognitive components found in competent physicians, my own assessment is that memory holds the upper hand.

In defining how much information one should memorize, Dr. Stead indicated that not only is extensive memorization a waste of time, but the human mind cannot retain an appropriate number of descriptors. Thus, he favored using computers instead of the human brain to store facts. This approach would allow physicians to concentrate their activity in organizing information and in thinking about the patient. Thus, his concept of a "Computerized Textbook of Medicine" was born. The salient feature of this resource was that pertinent information regarding the multiple descriptors of a given patient could be organized in a way that far surpassed the ability of an individual to remember all of these facts. This formulation is quite correct. The Duke Cardiovascular Databank, a "chapter" in Stead's vision of a "Computerized Textbook of Medicine," contains an enormous amount of patient-specific information. However, it was never tapped to provide useful, immediately available clinical information on a given patient. Why? Two possibilities: 1) the physicians were too hardheaded to use the data, or 2) no useful mechanism of organizing and making the information readily available was ever achieved. In fact, both factors played a role. Thus, at least at DUMC, the practice of cardiology was, and is, dependent on the individual physician's undoubtedly faulty memory of prior patients. Imperfect information, buttressed by an extensive knowledge of clinical trials (many of which apply only imperfectly to the patient in question), are the primary data used by the cardiologist in caring for patients.

Recently, the Internet has provided ready access to an enormous fund of general knowledge regarding medicine, and has added a wealth of useful information, which is available in the care of patients. Thus, a 21st century learner has a lot of general data on the pathophysiology and treatment of disease processes. Whether this has resulted in developing better physicians is a moot point. Personally, I am very dubious.

Information: Using It

Although the title, "Thinking Ward Rounds," would imply that a good deal of thought took place during Dr. Stead's attending rounds, from my vantage point, memorization was stressed—actually, not only stressed but demanded! The resident or student presenting a case to Dr. Stead had better damn well have memorized all the facts, important or not, regarding the patient's history, physical evaluation, laboratory work, prior laboratory work and everything else relating to the patient.[3] The information had to be between the "presenter's ears" and not read from a piece of paper. Thus, at least for the practical situation, little time was allocated for thinking either while preparing for, or during, ward rounds. The post-presentation critique of the patient's care frequently involved pointing out errors in the history or physical examination. Thinking about this information as it related to the need for further diagnostic or therapeutic approaches did not occupy a major portion of the time allocated, and fostering the development of clinical judgment by thinking was not stressed. It is true that, in contrast to most of his contemporaries, Dr. Stead's attending rounds eschewed a textbook type of review of the diagnosis and therapy of the suspected disease. We were expected to know the information in the "good books," but regurgitation of these data was not in order. What was demanded was that we commit to memory as many facts as possible about the patient. This information allowed the house officer to develop the clinical judgment necessary to assure that the patient received optimal care.

The Attributes of a Good Doctor

How important is good clinical judgment (based on factual information) in the makeup of a competent physician? Several years ago, a number of Duke's former Chief Residents ranked the the various characteristics that define a "good doctor." This exercise was presented in 2005 at a symposium entitled "Strategies for Medical Education in the Department of Medicine at DUMC."[4] Our former Chief Residents evaluated the relative importance of three salient components — clinical judgment, responsibility and humility — that the American Board of Internal Medicine deemed important in the makeup of a good physician.

An elaboration of these three components would seem to be in order. The need for good clinical judgment, stemming from a sound base of knowledge and experience is relatively obvious. (Furthermore, outstanding excellence in technical skills is a must, if required by the individuals' subspecialty.) Responsibility requires acceptance of one's role as the patient's physician and the willingness to deal with the multiple issues that arise from fulfilling this role. In addition, a major component implicit in the definition of responsibility is a large serving of caring. A good doctor must like people and be motivated to do whatever is necessary to care for their needs. Humility was defined by the noted philosopher, Dirty Harry: "A man's got to know his limitations." Thus, a good doctor must have a sense of what he does and does not yet know. Implicit in this situation is a willingness to seek help from more knowledgeable experts. The doctor must recognize when a decision is based on a less than firm foundation and then be willing to change directions if dictated by the clinical situation. Indecisiveness is never the answer, but pig-headed adherence to an arbitrary course of action must be avoided.

The importance of these attributes was ranked by the 60 former Chief Medical Residents in terms of their relative contribution to good doctoring: clinical judgment 43% (range 28–75%), responsibility 34% (range 10–75%) and humility 23% (range 5–40%). Although it is obvious that there was a considerable range for each attribute, the largest number felt that clinical judgment was the most important. However, responsibility was also deemed of very high importance. My own assessment is that responsibility should have been paramount.

I believe that indoctrinating the trainee in the essential trait of responsibility was Dr. Stead's primary goal during his teaching rounds. By any criterion, Dr. Stead excelled at producing excellent physicians. Perhaps his most important contribution was the ability to motivate the trainee to function as a doctor. He employed the two mentoring tools, carrot and stick, but the latter predominated. The "take-home-message" from interactions with Dr. Stead, both on ward rounds and elsewhere, was that the key component of physician competence is responsibility. Dr. Stead's trademark admonition, "What this patient needs is a doctor," was most frequently employed because of a trainee's failure to fulfill the role of responsibility toward the patient, not a failure of cognitive function.[5]

How did Dr. Stead accomplish the task of indoctrinating responsibility? Certainly, he personally possessed the attributes of an excellent physician, but was by no means as encyclopedic in knowledge as were many of his contemporaries. So that emulating Dr. Stead as a fountain of knowledge was not, at least in my opinion, a worthwhile experience. Ward rounds with Dr. Stead, while informative, were not really designed for thinking but involved indoctrinating responsibility as the primary focus. Assuming responsibility for the patient was the quintessential component of the learning process under his tutelage. That this lesson was clearly understood by the house officer is exemplified by the invariable identification of the sick individual as "my patient"—never as a "case" of some disease or by some other descriptor. In my opinion, the difficulty currently found in medical education primarily stems from a lack of such direct identification with the responsibility for patients.

The Attention Concentrator

We must ask ourselves the question: What are the primary factors that strengthen or facilitate the process of learning to be a physician? One characteristic of attending rounds with Dr. Stead permeated all the participants: fear. I believe fear is a very powerful motivating force in learning. As Dr. Samuel Johnson so eloquently expressed, "Depend on it, sir. When a man knows he is to be hanged in a fortnight, it concentrates his mind wonderfully."[6] Personally, I believe Dr. Stead's attending rounds had all the characteristics of an imminent hanging. Fear of disapproval by Dr. Stead, or fear of looking ridiculous in front of one's peers, drove trainees to perform to their maximum ability. Is "Thinking Trumps Memorization" the primary lesson taught by Dr. Stead? No! Responsibility for the patient was the message.

Conclusion

In putting all of this together under the rubric of this treatise, my general assessment is as follows:

1. The concept that thinking is more important than memorization in developing the clinical judgment of a physician is false—learning is a "no trump" process.
2. Responsibility is the key component of good doctoring.
3. Dr. Stead was superior in motivating young physicians to develop responsibility.
4. The primary mechanism whereby he was so effective was that he "scared-the-hell" out of everybody with whom he came in contact!

References

1. *The American Heritage Dictionary of the English Language.* Fourth Edition, Boston/New York: Houghton Mifflin Company; 2000.

2. Stead EA Jr. *A Way of Thinking: A Primer on Being a Doctor.* Haynes BF (ed). Durham, N.C.: Carolina Academic Press; 1995.

3. Laszlo J, Neelon FA. *The Doctors' Doctor.* Durham, NC; Carolina Academic Press; 2006.

4. Strategies for Medical Education in the Department of Medicine at DUMC. Chief Medical Residents Society Reunion; October 2005.

5. Wagner GS, Cebe B, Rozear MP. (Eds). E.A. Stead Jr. *What This Patient Needs is a Doctor.* Durham, NC. Carolina Academic Press; 1978.

6. Boswell J. *The Life of Samuel Johnson.* Hibbert C (ed). Harmondsworth, Middlesex, UK: Penguin Books; 1979.

Comments Following "Thinking Trumps Memorization"

Bill Stead: I totally agree with Joe Greenfield's idea that the fundamental element of my father's teaching program was responsibility. But I wonder whether my father would actually characterize Jack Myers as the greatest physician. My father thought Jack was the greatest human computer, had the best fact base and an ability to focus that fact base on a patient, on a diagnosis. On the other hand, he said that if Jack was walking across a room and walked into a chair he would walk through it instead of walking around it. And my guess is that the best physician would connect with the obstruction in the room well enough to walk around it.

The other thing concerns memorization. That was a technique to let novices begin to recognize patterns, which is part of clinical judgment. I remember making rounds with him when I was an intern on Long Ward. Two patients with pneumonia were admitted to me one night, and I got mixed up about which one had the high white blood cell count and which one, low. My father made it extremely clear that to not know who had the low white count was to miss the most important thing that would identify who was really going to do poorly if I didn't do something fast. Pattern recognition is the clue to whether *this* patient is sick.

Mort Bogdonoff: Dr. Greenfield has hit the nail on the head. No one awaited Gene's arrival with a sense of utter ease. Over the years, I had the opportunity to create a friendship with him, but the very idea of calling him "Gene" didn't happen until I was forty. It took time to break through that sense of his being the master, and you had better man the lines of the ship very well.

Ruth Ballweg: I want to make four points. The first one has to do with memorization, with how people are usually told that they need to remember "medical" things because they are what is important. But in the example we heard earlier (see page 22), Dr. Whalen pointed out that Dr. Stead was concerned about the patient's psychosocial history. Dr. Stead was worried about what would happen because the patient was the "glue" that held her family together. I think that's the sort of thing we are losing because of our fixation with time. When people feel they don't have time, the attending physician may say, "I don't want to hear about that psychosocial stuff," or "Make that quick because we have to move ahead." When I hear about Dr. Stead, I love hearing about the psychosocial piece.

My second point has to do with our concern about the students of today. I show my students a movie called "The Making of a Physician," about medical education at Harvard. It depicts an older physician teaching on ward rounds very much like Dr. Stead did. My young students get very angry about that. They feel the doctor is harassing the students, that that kind of teaching is inappropriate and disrespectful, and should be reported to the dean of the medical school. I personally think it is funny, but people in their 20's and 30's have a hard time relating to this sort of tough love. Their criticism is not my criticism, but it's one that I hear people talking about.

I also wanted to mention the concepts of teams, which fits very well with Dr. Stead's point of view. With teams you delegate to people's strengths and you teach to people's weaknesses. You don't just take the team as it is, you constantly build the team up so that people are learning the things they don't know, and even the master teacher might learn something from a student.

Finally, I want to tell you a story about responsibility. I just came in from an around-the-world trip, and my bag got lost in Singapore. At the United Airlines office in Seattle, this wonderful person said, "Oh, let me find it for you." Two days later my bag came, and I was happy. The next day, I got a phone call saying, "This is United Air-lines. We want to find out about your bag and if you're happy you got it." I said, "Yes, and I want to thank the person who helped me." And he said, "Well, I'm that one, and I'm calling to tell you a story. Your card said you were a physician assistant and director of the PA program. I found your bag because two years ago I had some very strange pain in my legs. I couldn't figure it out. I went to the clinic and the PA there diagnosed a very unusual kind of cancer. It was a very subtle diagnosis. And they used the whole system to save my life. That PA took responsibility for my care from beginning to end, and that's been my experience in this primary care system I am in, so I'm calling to thank you for that. I found your bag because your student took responsibility and really demonstrated what responsibility in primary care means."

John Laszlo: I thought Dr. Greenfield's talk was right on, and his point of view seemingly in contrast to some of today's previous talks. But I don't think it really is. Most of us would probably admit there is a "tough love" aspect to medical training; it was certainly part of our training. Still there are a couple of paradoxes. Those of you who have read *The Doctors' Doctor* know that Gene Stead himself was, in many ways, scared of his own shadow as he was growing up. When I interviewed him, he talked about his various fears, and how he would maneuver to avoid people in authority. Given that, how did he manage to inflict such stress on his students? That seems to me one of Stead's paradoxes.

Another relates to the memory issue. During his years of school-ing — high school, college, medical school — he had no worries be-cause he knew he could get an "A" every time simply by memorizing the night before the test (he did, however, recognize that the "learn-ing" didn't last long). All this is downplayed when we talk about the value of thinking and the unimportance of memory. Maybe Joe could talk about how he dealt with memorization in his later life.

Joe Greenfield: I am not sure I can add very much. Probably each of us in this room saw Dr. Stead as a different person; we take our picture of him, if you will, and relate it back to our selves. So it's hard for me to look at Dr. Stead and what he meant to me, and deal with this whole memorization-versus-thinking issue because that's not what I remember him telling us. It seems pretty obvious that if you spend all your time memorizing and not thinking you would not turn out to have good clinical judgment. But in my experience, people who really have a lot of facts are able to put them together (I'm still trying to deal with the Jack Myers issue that Bill raised). Dr. Stead said about a lot of people on the faculty, "If there was a column in the middle of the room, this particular person, would run into it rather than walk around it. But that's got very little to do with whether he was a good doctor or not."

Robert Klein, MD, Emeritus Professor of Medicine at the University of Rochester School of Medicine and Dentistry, has "always been interested in the borderland between medicine and psychiatry; Eugene Stead helped me learn that was my area":

I've made some notes related to both this morning's session as well as this afternoon's. I spent 39 years in Rochester, New York, but before that I had come to Duke from Alabama in 1954 as a senior medical student. John Burnham, who had been to Duke, suggested I come, so I took senior medicine and fell under the influence of Dr. Stead and Mort Bogdonoff. When I came back for my internship and residency, I remember that Dr. Stead and one of the professors from psychiatry conducted what was called the Patient Care Conference—a weekly, one-hour session during which a patient from one of the wards was presented, and the nuances of the patient's illness discussed by Dr. Stead and the psychiatrist together. Each had a lot of respect for each other, and that was really where I became interested in what, at that time, was called psychosomatic medicine. I took a fellowship under Mort Bogdonoff, which encouraged my interest in the relationship between psychiatry and medicine. Then George Engel, whose brother, Frank was at Duke, visited and talked about his program in Rochester. He enticed me to go up there for a two-year fellowship in what was then called medical-psychiatric liaison (this mind/body business has suffered through a lot of name changes over the decades). I learned in

Rochester what Engel later wrote up as the "biopsychosocial model of disease." Looking back, I think that's the model that Stead worked with and which kept him interested in all the dimensions of the patients on rounds, in all the relationships and psychosocial interactions that set the stage for stress and illness. I think Stead operated in that model, although George Engel really developed it and wrote about it at Rochester.

I also want to mention that Dr. Stead arranged for Dr. Bingham Dai, the lay psychoanalyst, to put Stead's chief residents through a year-long psychosocial inventory so they would begin to understand themselves better as people. I think that, too, reflected Stead's deep commitment to the biopsychosocial model.

Now I am 79 and retired, but I still teach the first-year medical students at Rochester. They've revised the curriculum to introduce the teaching of clinical skills in the first year. Those students also go to physician's offices for ambulatory experience. I teach them interviewing and physical examination; then, after they've been in the doctor's offices, they come back and we review the details of a patient that they have seen in the primary care practice. And when they present to me, they had better know a lot about the person, not just their symptoms and their blood pressure. I insist that they talk about the patient as a person, even though the patient isn't there in front of us. I think that's the key to staying interested in the patient.

B. W. Ruffner, MD, recently stepped down from being Interim Dean of the Chattanooga unit of the Tennessee Medical School and is now President-Elect of the Tennessee Medial Association:

I am a medical oncologist in Chattanooga who's been teaching since I left Duke. A very significant distinction about memorization that hasn't been emphasized enough is this: Earl Metz stayed up all night to make sure that he knew everything possible about the patient he was to present the next day. This is very different than staying up all night to memorize a textbook. As I remember, Dr. Stead made it very clear that he thought all exams should be open book tests. There is too much stuff that we don't need to cram into our brains.

Britain W. Nicholson, MD, is Chief Medical Officer and Senior Vice President of the Massachusetts General Hospital:

I'm an internist and an administrator, who's been in Boston for 30 years. Before that I was a medical student and house officer at Duke, and had the good fortune of having a one-on-one tutorial with Dr. Stead during a year I spent in an outreach program at the Oxford Hospital north of Durham. I want to address two items that have come up today.

In my experience, despite Dr. Stead's influence on a number of people including those in this room, his method of teaching was the exception rather than the rule at Duke. One question today asked, "What's the appropriate format for attending rounds?" I would change this a little and say, "What's the appropriate setting for attending rounds?" Every system is perfectly designed to achieve the results that it gets. Look at what's happened with inpatient medicine. Dr. Greenfield made the point earlier that we now have an 80-hour work rule for our residents. The second thing is that over 85% of patients are admitted to the hospital under the strictures of prospective reimbursement, so the incentives all push for short admissions. And thirdly, over the years, the gap between payments for Evaluation and Management services and payments for procedural services has grown and grown. So there is certainly less emphasis on E&M activities, which makes it extraordinarily difficult to achieve the learning and teaching style that Dr. Stead exercised during his years on the wards. I agree entirely with what Harvey Cohen said earlier: we've got to move teaching to other settings, especially the outpatient setting, but we shouldn't confuse methods with values. Dr. Stead's values, his patient-centered teaching, which I think we all actually embrace, doesn't have to depend on the method by which it is achieved. We always did it in the inpatient setting, and we shouldn't abandon the wards, but that shouldn't be the exclusive setting.

In terms of how the attending physician can facilitate the development of clinical judgment and responsibility, I couldn't endorse more what Bill Stead said several times this morning, and Joe Greenfield reiterated, about the responsible physician. In my experience with Dr. Stead, both on Osler Ward and during my year-long tutorial, he never left any doubt that that patient in front of me was *my* responsibility; *I* had to be the advocate for that patient. That sort of teaching only comes from somebody whose orientation differs entirely from somebody who acts as a consultant, who feels that their only responsibility is to put out information for you to accept or reject. Modeling responsibility is extraordinarily important.

K. Patrick Ober: I think it is a little artificial to set memorization opposite thinking. My guess is that Dr. Stead assumed memorization, assumed that people had facts and if they didn't have them, by God, they were going to go get them. I learned that when he was a medical student there was some question as to whether he was going to pass one course, not because he didn't know stuff but because he didn't go to lectures. He didn't go because it was a waste of time— he could read a book and learn in five minutes whatever the lecturer was going take an hour to explain. My guess is that owning medical facts was, for him, very much a given thing. If you're going to be a good doctor you're going to have to know a whole lot of facts, but the time that you had with him would be time spent on how you use those facts, how you apply those facts. It would be an interesting exercise for everybody who actually worked with Dr. Stead to write down the most important fact that they learned from him. My guess would be there would either be a whole lot of facts or none at all. I think what Dr. Stead taught was not facts; he taught himself as a person, as an individual, as someone with standards. He taught responsibility. He taught accountability. He taught commitment.

Hal Silberman: Gene Stead was an accurate physician in terms of physical exam, but one of the important things he did was to think out loud on rounds. In a recent paper (Lancet. 2007;370:705–11), Brendan Reilly notes importantly that clinical medicine is messy. The beginning of formulating a differential diagnosis is messy, even chaotic sometimes. Stead was brave enough to go through that. Many clinicians don't want to expose themselves so they don't (or can't) think out loud. But thinking out loud on rounds may be one of the important ways that an attending physician can facilitate the development of clinical judgment and responsibility. If you challenge someone with a question, "How do you teach somebody?" it's frightening. Jeff Wong said he's not sure that we can teach teachers to be better teachers; he doesn't know yet. I would tell him what George Engel said to me once, when I was in charge of the Patient Care conference that I inherited from Mort Bogdonoff, and was referred to today by Bob Klein. I said I didn't know how to teach what I was doing and Engel said, "Well, you better find out right away or stop doing it." And I really never could find out how to teach it, other than take the history from a very difficult and troubled patient in front of other learners—and do it with a touch of kindness.

Mike McLeod: In advocating for the patient, we bring compassion and our skills, and yet the final choice is the patient's. The patient must decide whether to follow our advice or not. I think that sometimes we physicians measure our success by whether the patient did what we said he should do, but that's an unfair measuring stick. I think we have to bring our best skills, be totally responsible, but realize that the patient may make a different choice for their own reasons. And we can still feel good about what we have brought to the interaction.

Willoughby Lathem, MD, retired and living in Connecticut, was a medical student and intern under Gene Stead at Emory and Grady Hospital in 1945–47, and a resident at Duke under Gene Stead from 1947–48:

I think I knew Dr. Stead well, and I've heard things of tremendous interest here today, but I have not heard mentioned Stead's extensive legacy beyond the field of clinical medicine. Take my own career as an example. After finishing all my training, I had a career in academic medicine, including six years with Jack Myers in Pittsburgh (and as an aside, Jack Myers was not the best physician I have ever known—Gene Stead was). After about 10 years, I changed careers and went into international health, which has let me visit over 90 countries and live in seven of them. This is a far cry from thinking and learning at the bedside, but nonetheless I have applied the principles that I learned under Stead to the work I have done around the world. His teaching of the power and method of observation, of analysis, of deductive reasoning, of thoughtful analysis has served me well in my long and now retired career. I even tried to apply those principles from time to time in my private life, but my wife did not appreciate it. In any event, I think what we have been discussing today, and the thoughts that we have articulated have wide application. Certainly my international work was a direct result of the years that I spent working and studying under Gene Stead.

Elizabeth Ross: I always come back to the education question. I look at memorization like I look at the ABCs: you have to learn the alphabet before you can know words, before you can write something, before you can put something together. Some things students just have to memorize, but at some point, like on rounds at the bedside, I say put the computer away, put the Blackberry away, and discuss the process of making a decision for this patient. Students often like to hide behind data, and there's so much data today that is easy to do. But to actually synthesize the data, to listen to a patient is different.

I think that students are sometimes reluctant to delve too deeply because they're not sure what they're going to get. If you listen to a patient talk, you get into emotion and other things that you're not sure how to handle. Like data, that can sometimes get in the way.

I have heard people say today, "We were really scared to death of Dr. Stead." I wonder about how to give feedback to students in a way that is conducive to learning. I'd like to get to the point that students are less afraid of disappointing the physician-mentor than of disappointing the patient; more afraid of failing their patient rather than failing the person who is guiding them.

Bud Shelton: In my association with Dr. Stead as a PA and as a close friend in his latter years, I don't remember him ever telling me he was disappointed in anything I said or did, but he could use those eyes and tell me the whole world. And I haven't heard too many people say much about his ears except that they're large, but I found Dr. Stead to be the ultimate listener. He was patient enough to listen to every word you said, in the order that you wanted to say it, and only rarely would he ask for some clarification. And it always amazed me how rapidly, after you poured your heart and soul out about some personal, or business, or medical matter, that he would ask a couple of questions, and pretty soon you had answered the question you had brought in the first place.

Bill Stead: As long as we are touching on the fear factor, I think it would probably be useful for people to know, as John Laszlo mentioned, that my father could be as afraid as anybody else. I did not appreciate this until my father was getting ready to receive the Kober medal from the Association of American Physicians. I found him rehearsing his presentation in the Washington Sheraton, and I can tell you his sphincter tone was tight.

I think, in essence, that he had an idea of responsibility, an idea of excellence, and each of us who wanted to perform to that level were afraid that we might not, and therefore we worked hard at trying to get to that level. I think that's one piece of it. I never found him to be a disciplinarian in the sense of beating up on you. What he would, in fact, do was force you to make up the deficit when he perceived that you had not done what you needed to do, or exercised your responsibility. He gave you the opportunity to do it.

Chapter 6

Brain Sorting in the 21st Century

Galen S. Wagner, MD

In his 1983 essay entitled "Brain Sorting," Eugene Stead wrote:

> The fact that differences in function define differences
> in structure is accepted and used by all students of med-
> icine for all organs except the brain. The complexity of
> human behavior, the complexity of the structural or-
> ganization of the brain, and the acceptance of the spirit
> and mind as attributes separate from the structure of
> the brain, have all tended to obscure the obvious —
> namely, that at any point in time the response of the
> brain to inputs is determined by its structure. By ob-
> serving the response to multiple inputs, brains can be
> sorted into a series of boxes, each box containing brains
> structurally more similar than those in the other boxes.[1]

We have recently celebrated the end of the 20th Century; and now
we celebrate the end of Dr. Stead's Century. At the beginning of
these centuries, the atom, the microbe, and the human brain were
all mysteries. But by mid century, split-atoms and antimicrobials
were limiting the capacities of wars and diseases to prematurely de-
stroy human lives; and schools were sorting pre-mature human
brains by IQ to provide the education required to thrive, rather
than only survive, through the maturity and even post-maturity
now available to them.

By mid 20th century Dr. Stead had arrived in the North Carolina Piedmont with his own brain sorted in the South (Atlanta), North (Boston), and West (Cincinnati). He was prepared to thrive in his maturity; and even the post-maturity that would almost complete a century of his own life. Dr. Stead's philosophy of education was built on the principle that the "ability to make high grades in school and excel in aptitude tests may not translate into an outstanding performance in our irrationally-run world. Performance is greatly modified by the non-IQ portion of our brains. The more persons touched in the course of the day, the more limiting becomes the non-IQ portion of the brain. I am performance-sensitive and examination-insensitive."[2]

Dr. Stead's philosophy of education had been formed through a sequence of experiences that had proceeded from home to community to school-room to laboratory to bed-side:[3]

- In the home, "we grew up thinking that if you wanted to get up in the morning and do something nobody could stop you."
- In the community, "The only times I ever won prizes were at the YMCA. I had the biggest ears and I could put on my shoes and socks faster than anyone else."
- In school, "I studied in high school because I found learning fun."
- In college, "I took biology because my sister's boyfriend pointed out that one particular assistantship was the best-paying undergraduate job on the campus."
- He chose Medical School, "Because it offered more intellectual challenge than any other area on my college campus."
- In the laboratory he "learned the importance of appreciating what is not known about a condition as well as what is known."
- At the patient's bedside, "Excellent performance has its own reward."
- After these many educational experiences Dr. Stead summarized the sorting of his own brain: "Just as many people like to fish or play golf, I like to work with my head."

The Nature of Brain Sorting

During the two decades of his maturity that spanned the middle of the 20th Century, Dr. Stead served as Chairman of the Duke Medical School Department of Medicine. During his final almost four decades, he shared the wisdom of his post-maturity in many ways, including his essay on "Brain Sorting." He begins by distinguishing the ways in which he and neurologists sort brains: "Neurologists sort brains of their patients when changes of structure which produce major defects in motor, sensory or autonomic functions have occurred. I, on the other hand, am interested in the sorting of brains when the neurologist reports a normal neurological examination."[4]

Dr. Stead explained his method: "I have been interested in what I call brain sorting: putting like brains into the same basket. Since the brains I dealt with were in live persons, I could not use anatomical techniques, but I knew that the brains with identical responses to a wide variety of inputs would be similar in structure, and that brains with a great divergence in outputs from my battery of inputs would be different. I could therefore sort brains into subgroups without knowing the precise anatomical configurations underlying the subgroups."[5]

Dr. Stead tells of the use of this brain-sorting method on his first experimental subject — himself. He had found that he was so tone deaf that, "On the day of the 1981 Kentucky Derby, ... I told my wife that ... the band was playing 'My Old Kentucky Home'! She rejoined that ... the band was playing 'The Star Spangled Banner.' I also have a relative deficit in recognizing form and shape. I cannot draw my wife's face. I have never known the color of anyone's eyes."[5]

Dr. Stead illustrates the contrast between brains sorted by their recognition of tone, form, shape, and color by comparing his brain to that of Georgia O'Keeffe who said: "'The meaning of a word — to me — is not as exact as the meaning of a color. Color and shapes make a more definite statement than words.' By contrast, when Gene Stead says a word, he forms a picture in [his] brain that is much more specific and concrete than the image imprinted on his brain when he sees a picture of the scene described by the word."[5]

Dr. Stead illustrates the "clinical significance" of his kind of brain-sorting by considering the "burden-lifting" effect on the parents of a child with dyslexia when they receive "the knowledge that these difficulties have an anatomical basis and are not caused by inter-personal relationships. Children who learn slowly in social situations do so because the inputs that create usual pictures in most people create different images in the brain of the slow social learner. These persons can be helped by teaching them to find out what the more average person has seen and then to correct their own pictures."[5]

Dr. Stead then explains how he sorted the brains of his later "experimental subjects," his Chief Medical Residents, by "offering them the opportunity of working with the distinguished Chinese psychoanalyst, Bingham Dai." In his Duke "clinical laboratory" — the Osler Ward bed-sides — Dr. Stead observed that, in the repetitive person-to-person reactions of these talented young physicians, they "behaved predictably, wasted a large amount of energy, became fatigued, and, as far as I could see, learned nothing about themselves or the persons with whom they were reacting." After a year of brain sorting therapy with Dr. Dai, "They came to accept their uniqueness. They realized that they were excellent in many areas but limited in others. They discovered that their brains limited their behavior and that brain changing was difficult."[5]

Brain Sorting in Education

By mid 20th Century, the American philosopher John Dewey had almost completed his own near-century of life that began in 1859. At the time of his death in 1952, the columnist Benjamin Fine observed that, "Fifty years ago education was based on the authoritarian principle that 'teacher knows best'. The subject was the most important part of the classroom — and the child the least important. Dewey believed that the school should keep alive and direct the active inquiring attitude of the child. Education in this country can never return to the pre-Dewey era, any more than science can return to the pre-atomic period, or medicine to the pre-penicillin days."[6]

The Dewey philosophy considered that "Education is not something to be forced upon youth from without, but is the growth of capacities with which human beings are endowed at birth." Brain sorting was essential to this enterprise because "The child's own interests and powers furnish the material and give the starting-point for all education."[7] And who would serve as "neuro-therapist" to guide this process? Dewey recognized that "The teacher is indeed more important than in the traditional system because it is more difficult to direct 'natural activities' along a coherent line of development than to follow a previously fixed program."[8] "Utilization of interest and habit to make [education] something fuller, wider, more refined and under better control, might be defined as the teacher's whole duty."[9]

The Stead philosophy of "what this patient needs is a doctor" considered that "each disease resides in a person; and just as diseases can be sorted and placed in categories, the brains of the persons with the diseases can be sorted."[5] Those of us fortunate enough to have been sorted into Dr. Stead's presence have dedicated our own professional lives to this "doctoring" responsibility in our own ways; and now we seek to carry our wisdom into the new century. As we accept the daunting responsibility of building a firm foundation for meeting the challenges of sorting the brains we encounter, we should remember Dr. Stead's principle that, "by observing the response to multiple inputs, brains can be sorted into a series of boxes, each box containing brains structurally more similar than those in other boxes."[1]

Just 10 years after John Dewey's death, the folk singer Malvina Reynolds complained in her song *Little Boxes* that "people all went to the university where they were put in boxes and they came out all the same, and there's doctors and lawyers and business executives, and they're all made out of ticky-tacky, and they all look just the same."[10] Although John Dewey's focus on, "the child's own interests as ... the starting-point for all education" may have equaled the "importance" of the atomic bomb and penicillin, it certainly has not achieved the permanent influence on education that the atom has in science or the antibiotic in medicine.

The late 20th century philosopher Mortimer Adler provides insight into why we have failed to develop "individual-focused education." Adler sorted human knowledge into 106 "Great Ideas," among which he included art, medicine, and education.[11] He wrote essays on each of these 106 ideas as the basis for his index of the Encyclopedia Brittanica's "Great Books" series, and then updated these concepts through Brittanica's annual "Great Ideas Today." He followed Aristotle in sorting art into "creative" and "cooperative" categories; and considered that the healing of medicine and the learning of education occur only when the physician or teacher cooperates with nature. Adler sorted education into the "intellectual virtues" of "knowledge, understanding and wisdom;" and then identified the "means" of achieving these ends as occurring through "telling facts, coaching skills, and discussing concepts," respectively.[12]

I had the opportunity to explore Adler's sorting of knowledge when I collaborated with Mark Swaim on the essay, "Rethinking the Art of Medicine" for the 1996 edition of The Great Ideas Today."[13] It became obvious that no sorting of patient's brains can occur in a medical system that reduces clinical diagnosis to technology-based "imaging" of organs, and no sorting of student's brains can occur in an education system that reduces teaching to lecture-based provision of not only facts, but also skills and concepts.

Mentoring as Brain Sorting

John Dewey said, "What the best and wisest parent wants for his own child, that must the community want for all of its children."[14] Before the Greek hero Ulysses left his home on the island of Ithaca to begin the Trojan War, he entrusted the education of his son, Telemachus, to his friend Mentor. Now, in the 21st century, "What this student—any student—needs is a wise mentor—many wise mentors." Unlike the teacher who "shows" and "instructs," the mentor, like the parent, follows Dr. Stead's method of "observing the response of each individual to multiple inputs."

In the Olympic Games that have spanned the past century, the heights and speeds and distances that won medals have climbed steadily upward. Gold medal winners in 1900 would not have even qualified to compete in 2008. This ever-increasing excellence in functions that are not the distinguishing capabilities of humans has been achieved by childhood sorting of both bodies and brains by coaches skilled as mentors. How can we apply this same method to achieve ever-increasing excellence in the thinking-to-solve-problems that is the primary human-distinctive capability? The 18th Century English philosopher John Ruskin in his essay, "A Tool or a Man" has stated "You can teach a man to draw a straight line, and to cut one; to strike a curved line, and to carve it ... with ... admirable speed and perfect precision; and you find his work perfect of its kind; but if you ask him to think about any of those forms, to consider if he cannot find any better in ... his own head, he stops; his execution becomes hesitating; he thinks, and ten to one he thinks wrong; ten to one he makes a mistake in the first touch he gives to his work as a thinking being. But you have made a man of him for all that. He was only a machine before, an animated tool."[15]

In my own career I also discovered that, like Stead, "I like to work with my head;" and so I have tried to develop my skills as a mentor. I coach the problem-solving required to design, perform, and publish clinical research. My success with each student depends on my ability to match my coaching to his or her own mind—that is, on "brain sorting." Although each student is unique, I must sort them into categories based on similarities.

The Myers-Briggs Personality Scale provides a model for sorting of the ways that brains prefer to focus their attention (introversion vs extroversion), take in information (sensing vs intuition), make decisions (thinking vs feeling), and orient toward the outer world (judging vs perceiving).[16] I have used this model to construct scales to sort other categories of brain function. These include: acceptance of criticism (open vs closed), need for a structured environment (guideline vs schedule), level of self-esteem (under- vs over-confident), and dependence on parental control (adolescent vs adult).

Dr. Stead provided a cardinal principle for brain sorting when he said that one of the characteristics of the "great teacher" is the ability to "create a shadowy framework in which the student can climb."[17] The student should be encouraged to discover a research subject of personal interest through the mentoring capabilities of their own conscious and sub-conscious minds. Dr. Stead further explains his concept: "If the teacher fills in the skeleton in great detail, he will limit the learning by his own knowledge. If he makes the form recognizable but leaves the final shape and details to the student, the student may produce a much better intellectual synthesis than the teacher. A teacher may be likened to an artist. A pedestrian artist may produce an exact copy of a scene and most viewers will see approximately the same thing. The picture will not live because it will have little relevance to the changing patterns of life. A much less precise picture, suggesting a mother and child which leaves many details to the imagination, will come to life in as many interpretations as there are viewers. Some of these interpretations may be superior to the original concept of the artist."[17]

What Does the Future Hold?

Dr. Stead provided another tool for brain sorting in his 1972 essay, *The Way of the Future*, in which he described his computerized textbook of medicine: "Computer science can change medical practice. Information can be collected and stored in a way that allows the doctor to use all of his experience to care for the patient—not just the portion he can remember.... The computer can carry many more subgroups in its memory than the doctor."[18] Similar technology could be used to build a "computerized textbook of education" to provide the data-banks of students sorted by their key brain characteristics and followed to document the outcomes of education interventions that could guide the mentoring of future students.

The emerging technologies that form the basis of "Cognitive Neuroscience" provide promise in this century for ever more precise brain sorting. Methods of creating ways of directly observing the responses of an individual's brain to multiple inputs will provide data to support the educational intervention decisions of future mentors. This will bring further fulfillment of Dr. Stead's method of filling his boxes with brains that are "structurally more similar than those in other boxes."[1]

References

1. Stead EA Jr. Brain Sorting. In *A Way of Thinking*. Haynes, B. (ed). Durham, NC: Carolina Academic Press. 1995, p.101.

2. Ibid. p.108.

3. Stead EA Jr. Each year I cheerfully send Emory a check. In Wagner G, Cebe B, Rozear M (eds). *What This Patient Needs Is a Doctor*, Durham, NC: Carolina Academic Press: 1981. pp.145–51.

4. Stead EA Jr. (1995). Op.cit. p.97.

5. Ibid. pp.106–108.

6. Fine B. "John Dewey's Great Influence on the Schools of America Weighed by Leading Educators." New York Times, June 8, 1952.

7. Dewey J. Schools of Tomorrow. New York: E.P. Dutton & Co, 1915.

8. Dewey J. *Democracy and Education*. New York: The Macmillian Co, 1916.

9. Dewey J. *Educational Essays*. London: Blackie & Son, 1910.

10. Reynolds, M. Little Boxes. In *The Malvina Reynolds Songbook*. Berkeley, CA: Schroder Music Company, 1962. pp.44–45.

11. Adler, M. *The Great Ideas*. MacMillian Publishing Company, New York, 1992.

12. Adler, M. The Same Course of Study for All. In Adler, M. (Ed.) *The Paedeia Proposal*, Macmillan Publishing Company, New York. 1982, p.23.

13. Swaim M, Wagner G. Rethinking the art of medicine. In Van Doren, J. (Ed.), *The Great Ideas Today*. Encyclopedia Britannica, Chicago, 1996, pp.50–84.

14. Dewey J. *The School and Society*. Chicago: The University of Chicago Press, 1900.

15. Ruskin J. *Selected Writings*. The Penguin Group, England, 1982

16. Isabel Briggs Myers. *Introduction to Type*. Consulting Psychologists Press, Palo Alto, CA. 1993.

17. Stead EA Jr. The limitations of teaching. Pharos. 1969;32:54–7.

18. Stead EA Jr. Presidential Address, Association of American Physicians. Trans Assoc Am Phys 1972;85:1.

Comments Following "Brain Sorting in the 21st Century"

Chuck Beauchamp: One way that Dr. Stead guided people was by demonstrating at the bedside the utter eloquence of creating a personalized solution for the patient. He pointed us towards that solution, in part by pointing out that the patients themselves often could come up with answers to our dilemmas. That provided a very big drive for me to go into primary care medicine. He also made us think about how much we didn't know. Harvey Estes alluded to the Pickwickian syndrome—I remember a grand rounds on Pickwickian syndrome where Stead basically told the chief resident that he didn't know what's going on if he was satisfied with saying only that the patient was obese; something else must be going on that we didn't understand and we should look into it. He was never satisfied with our first answers; he always pushed us to go further than what we already knew about a particular situation.

Jeff Wong: Brain sorting can be applied to helping learners figure out what careers they should pursue. I'm working now with beginning level medical students—the ultimate multipotent stem cell, as it were. They haven't differentiated into anything yet, and many external factors determine the careers that they choose. Obviously, there is the money issue. When I decided to go into primary care, it wasn't very much in vogue and it still isn't. We're still struggling with how to get people to want to do that, but I think it boils down to brain sorting. Maybe personality profiles like the Myers-Briggs, or other ways of sorting students, could help us figure it out. I try to sort my students by offering different dichotomies: Are you a person who enjoys working with your hands or someone who enjoys working with you mind, as Dr. Stead said of himself.

Lois Flaherty: I have one caveat. This does smack a little bit of determinism. In the education field, children get sorted on the basis of some presumed characteristics that may or may not turn out to be valid. We don't know enough about whether people can change their ways of functioning and thinking and learning to be able to say, right from the beginning, that this one belongs in this category or that one in that category. This seems to me an important area for investigation, but we must be wary of the danger of premature closure.

Galen Wagner, MD, a resident under Stead in 1965–67 and thereafter a faculty member in his department, became Director of the Duke Coronary Care unit in 1968; under Stead's mentorship, he developed the Duke Internal Medicine Commmunity Outreach Program; in collaboration with Andy Wallace he directed the Cardiology Fellowship Program and developed the Duke Cardiovascular Fellowship Society; with Joe Greenfield he developed the Stead Scholarship Program and DUCCS, the Duke University Cooperative Cardiovascular Society:

I'd like to respond to Lois, because in thinking through Dr. Stead's essay I moved from believing I could sort brains to how I might help people to sort themselves. Rather than putting sorted brains into a box and then closing the lid, the mentor helps learners do an internal sorting, to figure out what really does drive them. As Jeff Wong just said, certain people seem to have always known what they wanted to do, but many others say they don't know. You know that they make choices, but those choices may be made subconsciously, and you though know they've made a choice, they just can't see that. They consciously believe, "I haven't figured out what I want to do," so they run around trying to get various people to tell them what they should do. I find myself helping to convince them that they really have it inside. They are moving to the drummer, and we have to help them realize what that cadence is.

Celeste ("Lessie") Robb-Nicholson, MD, a Duke medical student a long time ago and now a practicing internist at Massachusetts General Hospital and Associate Professor at Harvard Medical School, is Editor-in-Chief of Harvard Women's Health Watch, and Associate Chief of the General Medicine Division at MGH; she knew Dr. Stead through the enthusiasm of his proteges, in particular, Dr. Galen Wagner, and her husband, Dr. Brit Nicholson:

I want to stick a little bit longer with this subject of how we sort out clinical information and teach that to students, because I think it is best taught by modeling. Adult learners who come to us as students have already done a ton of information sorting throughout their education, and at the end of the day it's up to them to make a decision. However, it helps to practice this sorting, and teaching around the patient in front of us is the place to practice it. We miss opportunities to teach in the Socratic way for many reasons: it's more comfortable to sit around a conference table, or talk in generalities and, often, we're afraid to expose our own thinking. My favorite beef is that attending rounds resemble the story of the emperor's new clothes — everyone nods their heads and agrees in a somewhat robotic manner. But do we consistently say why we ask a question or make an assertion, and thereby expose our own thinking?

I didn't know Dr. Stead personally, but what I see of the way he taught was that students and the professor were on the same side together, solving the patient's problem. And if I expose my thinking and make it safe for students to expose their thinking, they begin to sort their own thoughts out. Every time ambulatory physicians, such as I am, whether in our office or attending on the in-patient service, are willing to say, "Why are we doing that? What is it we know? What do I know? What do you know? How do we put it together?" we help adult learners begin to understand their ways of thinking. The bedside with the patient is one of the very best vehicles for this, and its right there in front of us. It's certainly not rocket science, but it takes discipline, time and humility. And it requires the learner and teacher to participate actively in the process.

I often recall the education symposium that you, Galen, and Bill Anlyan organized many years ago at Duke. We talked about learning, and in the prepared readings, you provided a quote from Mortimer Adler that said, "There are three cooperative arts: farming, teaching and doctoring. These are arts that rely on a second element — the weather, the soil, the learner, or the patient." He felt that teaching and doctoring were similar processes, that we could use what we knew about teaching to be better doctors and what we knew about doctoring to be better teachers and learners. This was perfect synergy.

John Laszlo: Because Dr. Stead was such an astute listener he was able to sort people out very effectively. When I came to Duke in 1959, the faculty of medicine had 28 members, and he knew them all. He knew people he could rely on and send students to, and others who should be avoided because they were weaker. He paid very close attention to his house staff, and if you think that he left it to chance to sort yourself out, you're probably mistaken. A lot of people who entered specialties did so after a consultation with Dr. Stead that was more directive than they may have realized at the time. Take the example of Dr. [Albert] Heyman. He related to me his experience at Emory: A syphilis epidemic was affecting Atlanta and Dr. Stead saw the opportunity to get some money to study syphilis. He got a hold of a batch of penicillin but he needed someone who would administer it. And here was Dr. Heyman, a young, undifferentiated, internist who was persuaded by Stead that he wanted to run a syphilology program. Later, when he needed a neurologist to study the complications of neurosyphilis, he talked to Dr. Heyman. Dr. Heyman didn't know much about neurology so Stead sent him to the Mass General for a year or so of training and he became the chief neurologist at Duke. People were influenced to move in one direction or another on the basis of having their brains sorted by Dr. Stead.

John Flaherty, MD, graduated from Duke University School of Medicine in 1967; he is now retired from his faculty position at Johns Hopkins Medical School:

I was a cardiologist at Hopkins for 25 years, now retired. Brain sorting really happened to me when I came to Duke as a medical student. I looked for role models and the first one I discovered was Madison Spach, who was the ultimate clinician scientist. He got me comfortable with the idea that you can be both a clinician and a researcher in a kind of balance. Then I came across Gene Stead on Osler rounds, and realized the true value of a physical diagnosis in solving a patient's problems. I just got so turned on that I realized internal medicine had to be where to start, and later on I evolved into a cardiologist. I can remember those experiences on Osler Ward, where Stead would sort of tear you down, and then build you back up again. He would allow you to cook in your own juice a little bit, but at the end of the day, he'd put his arm around your shoulder and say, "Don't worry, you're going to become a fine doctor."

Ruby Wilson, EdD, RN, FAAN, Professor of Nursing and Dean, Emerita, of the Duke School of Nursing and assistant to the Chancellor for Health Affairs, was the first clinical nurse specialist at Duke; she had many opportunities to interact with Eugene Stead beginning in 1955 and extending beyond his retirement:

I came to Duke in 1955 and, of course, met Gene Stead. I was teaching senior [nursing] students in the new BSN program, and those students were included on Dr. Stead's teaching rounds on Osler Ward. However, unlike many who today have commented on how scared and intimidated they were, I never ever had that experience. Perhaps it was because I wasn't within the medical lineage responsible to him. I really think it would be a travesty, even though this symposium is directed toward physicians and PAs, not to recognize his legacy with nursing at Duke and, as a result of that, with nursing nationally and internationally.

Shortly after I arrived, Thelma Ingles and I talked about developing a masters program in clinical nursing because there was no such thing. At that time, all the masters programs in nursing aimed to produce administrators, teachers or supervisors, so Thelma and I came up with the idea of a clinical masters that would provide for specialization. Dr. Stead thought it was a good idea, so Thelma spent a year being mentored by him, after which we decided to move ahead with the experimental program. Of course, Gene always said, "You have to have money, too," and the Rockefeller Foundation provided support to the masters program for five years. Dr. Mort Bogdonoff subsequently became involved with us, and really supported the program, bringing a very important element of psychosomatic medicine to the implementation of the program. We admitted five students (four were graduates of Duke's new BSN program) in 1957, and they had experiences in various medical subspecialties (gastroenterology, cardiology, dermatology, etc). The

National League for Nursing (NLN) did not initially accredit this program, but after Thelma and I visited other top nursing schools and they developed clinical masters programs based on our model, the NLN did accredit it. This model then went international.

In looking at ways we could improve patient care, we responded to 16 graduating seniors, who wanted to provide nursing care the way they had been taught, and not the way they saw other nurses providing it. This was the start of the Hanes Project, and again Dr. Stead was very supportive of the idea. We moved into Hanes Ward for a year to focus on the patient/nurse/doctor relationship. Dr. Stead, always pointing out the need to have money, said, "You need to charge for the additional nursing care you're giving on that unit, because you're going to have 16 graduate nurses and you have to pay their salaries." I do believe it is the only time that nursing care was directly charged for at Duke, and the only time that nursing had money in its own coffers. We experimented with various approaches to nursing care, including having nurses' orders written on the same sheet as doctors' orders, and having nurses' observations entered chronologically with the doctors' progress notes. Dr. Stead and his medical staff supported those efforts and recognized the improved care on Hanes Ward. During this year, Dr. Stead invited me to attend his 9:00–9:30 AM Morning Report session with the two residents assigned to the private medical wards. This was considered a sacrosanct time by the residents and I know they wondered why Dr. Stead invited a nurse to share it.

Then I became the first clinical nurse specialist at Duke (in nephrology) with triad appointments in the School of Nursing, the School of Medicine, and the Nursing Services of the hospital. Dr. Stead one day asked if I would be willing to take some former military medical corpsmen into the dialysis program to see what I could teach them. Out of that experience the PA program was born. I won't go into all the details of how except to say that Dr. Stead was not happy with the School of Nursing because the faculty refused to develop a nurse practitioner (NP) program. Many of them thought that, as a clinical nurse specialist, I was practicing more medicine than nursing, and Dr. Stead became quite angry with nursing faculty, most of whom were women, because of the decision not to develop an NP program. So when we began to look at qualifications for admission to the PA program, Dr. Stead was unwilling to admit women. I was the only woman in the room with 10 other physicians, and I told him he had to admit women. He said, "No, I don't," and I said, "Well, if you don't want to admit women then I won't help you with the program," and walked out (I learned only later that no one ever disagreed with Dr. Stead in public or walked out on him!). The next day he called and said, "Well, Ruby, you won." I said, "What did I win?" He said, "Well, I decided we will admit women; now will you help me." Now when I see women PAs, I say, "You owe your position to me."

Back to the business of sorting brains. Gene thought that I would make a good doctor, so he had me admitted to the School of Medicine. When he told me about it, I was very upset. I told him it was not appropriate for him to make career decisions for me, and I did not appreciate it one bit. He said, "Well, I just think you'd make a damn good doctor." Ike Robinson, who overheard the interaction, came out of his office after Dr. Stead left, and said, "I never heard anybody talk to Dr. Stead the way you did and you even called him Gene!" I said, "He calls me Ruby." The next day, Dr. Stead came back and said, "Well, Ruby, I thought about what you said to me last night, and I've come to apologize. You are right. I'm wrong. It is your decision to decide what you want to be. Even so, you're still admitted to the School of Medicine. It's up to you whether you appear in the fall." And I said, "Well, I accept your apology, and I'm glad you see it my way. I hope we'll continue to be friends." So when you talk about brain-sorting, yes, I did have to sort within myself: I decided that a nurse was what I wanted to be and that is what I continue to be. However, I do value the many learning interactions I had with Dr. Stead, both the clinical moments associated with patient care and those of a more philosophical nature. He was a most insightful, serious, but also humorous man.

Hal Silberman: This business of replacing robotic responses with creative thinking is with us now and very demanding. I like to consider myself a student of Margaret Mead. I love to interact with patients and people. I find all kinds of behavior fascinating even if the individual is vomiting on my shoes in the ER. I have read the notes and charts of a great many physicians trained in other countries, who are here practicing a medicine so rigid that it terrifies me. If we were going to do something important, we better learn how to help them replace robotic responses with creative thinking because these individuals, like all of us, shape the opinion of humanity about doctors and doctoring.

And we need to sort out those who shouldn't be in medicine at all. Great teachers make a relationship with learners whereby they can say to one: "You did a terrible job today and the reason I know it is, I know you're capable of better. This is not sufficient, and must not happen again." Even greater teachers can reach the conclusion that this very expensive product, almost finished, doesn't belong in medicine. I don't know of anybody who's done that. I don't have a colleague who's taken a senior medical student aside and said, "You really are in the wrong field."

Bill Stead: I just made a list of things I have not yet heard spoken that are important parts of my father's teaching legacy. First, I think he was really the mind behind, and the person that got the decisions made for Duke's 1966 "New Curriculum" that, in essence, took out half the time devoted to memorizing facts and opened up room for basic research. I asked him how he was able to do that, and he said there was a brief window when the decision-making was concentrated in five people's hands and the Chairman of Surgery said, "Gene, you're interested in education. I'm not. You can have my vote." He needed only one more vote to get that fairly radical change made. When I asked him why the program hadn't been replicated, he said nobody else has been able to get a decision group small enough to do it. It is the best example of recognizing that we're better off teaching some people in depth than always going for breadth. Another thing that the New Curriculum did was to take a year of debt out of the system since most of the third year students get funded doing a year's research. So if we want to fix problems, we don't want to say our problem is there's not enough time, or we've got too many requirements from Washington; we need to think of some of these kinds of changes.

My second point concerns the PA program. Instead of requiring the clinical person who cares for the patient and takes responsibility for the patient be someone who's been through a long medical-educational process, we can take a person who has proven by experience that they can care for patients. We can give them enough education to do the job and be responsible, and thereby improve the care people get and decrease the cost.

One thing that he was not able to do was to get whatever classroom part of medical education is going to survive out of the expensive infrastructure of the medical school, and get it either online or into undergraduate colleges. We don't need expensive infrastructure for that part. Moving it out would decrease the cost, and every time we take down the cost, we take down debt and free up money for something else.

Finally, I think he was convinced that it was important to use simulation for teaching technical skills, not for thinking. I suspect that if he were here, he would be asking us to think radically. The principles we've discussed (and I think we agree that these principles are as valid today as they ever were) need some radical new approaches that will let us deliver those principles in today's environment.

Chapter 7

Teachers of Medicine and Their Students

Harold R. Silberman, MD

Picture this: a New Yorker magazine cartoon, perhaps from the 1970s; a young child's most innocent face looks up at an obviously professorial individual sitting in a large overstuffed leather chair reading a thick tome, presumably one of the many volumes along a wall of books behind and to either side of said reader. The youngster, from his perch on his haunches, requests: "Teach me something I'll remember the rest of my life!" This cartoon illustrates several different aspects of teaching and learning, including the teachable moment as well as the questions: Do we teach? Does the student learn what we teach or learn because we teach? Is teaching and learning part of a scheme wherein each actor knows his role but succeeds or fails independent of any inherent relationship?

Eugene Stead never believed in the idea that learning occurred because someone was teaching. Indeed, he feared that teachers interfered with learning! He devoted more than one session late in his life to the concept that we don't need teachers. After all, we have rapid access to up-to-date facts by simply, in his words, "Googling" them on the internet. At one of those sessions I held to the opposite view; namely, that we need teachers even on rounds—perhaps especially on rounds—where we may have a "great" patient with so much going on that the learner does not know where to start or what questions to ask about the case, or worse yet, does not even know what questions have been raised by the history, physical exam, and the initial laboratory data. In other words, there is too much to learn and one needs a guide, someone to help discard chaff that arises while threshing the wheat. In addition, the teacher can help the learner avoid going too far afield, which can happen when one sign or symptom might belong to several diseases and only by selecting from among facts can one make a diagnosis that fits like a glove. Then, there is the more serious aspect of the debate, namely, the value of having someone very close by, who can answer several of the simple questions early and thereby move the discussion to a more appropriate plane. Does the learner have to look up everything, even when it can be done so easily with an electronic library? This question may be the key one in any debate about how to teach and how/when to learn.

More likely than not, Dr. Stead knew the answer to most of his tough questions because he opined all those many years that great teachers didn't need to know all the answers; rather they needed to ask great questions—that is, make the student think for his grade.

The Tyranny of Time

Ultimately, time must factor into our considerations. For example, how much time can (or should) be allotted to analyzing a given patient's illness? This factor has always been a matter of practicality, and sometimes of urgency, especially when dealing with true emergencies. Today, of course, time limits are set by length of stay, by the duration of too-brief outpatient clinic visits, by the economic facts of life, and even more strictly by the Accreditation Council for Graduate Medical Education (ACGME), which specifies duty hours of learners in the hospital inpatient setting. The result is a clash of concepts presented to the learner: "Here, take on this patient with many complex problems, one or more of which could be in exacerbation and causing havoc with several systems. Learn what you can from talking with her or him while (s)he is an acutely ill historian; learn what is happening to the patient's body and physiology by a physical examination that yields too many clues; modify your impression by serial physical examinations plus

monitoring, as well as by initial laboratory data and imaging studies. Then fine-tune your diagnosis and plan of therapy by further
laboratory testing, the results of which require that there be several more tomorrows in your relationship with this patient. Oh,
and by the way you cannot carry out this task as an isolated exercise inasmuch as you have other patients whose physical status may
be getting worse either because of your treatment plan or in spite
of it."

Intuitively, we all know that learning of the kind we want to fos-
ter takes time, and that only parts of it can be gleaned from care shared
with a colleague. Continuity of care by a single physician for a given
patient may be labor-intensive but is usually the best approach both
to care and to learning, although sometimes we will have to substitute a second method such as on-call/off-call/electronic sign out.
My premise, in part because of the system in which I learned to
practice medicine, is that if at all possible, continuous or mini-
mally interrupted care is the best way to teach, learn, and make
sick folk better. Given a choice, patients prefer it by far. Unfortunately, it is, in all likelihood, the most expensive in terms of time
commitment, at least for the learner and the teacher.

Eugene Stead's Philosophy of Learning

Back to Dr. Stead and my recollection of one of the important
principles that he reiterated over the years. I once heard him say:
"As long as the student is attached to a sick patient and what the student is doing is for the sick patient, then learning is taking and will
take place, which is not a waste of or abuse of the student's time."

Unfortunately, I see no way to go back to the old systems that
were once in place at Duke and at most other institutions of higher
medical education. It might be feasible, with heroic investment of
time and extraordinary expense of money on postgraduate medical
education, to increase the number of teachers who could spend
even more time perhaps than the house officers with whom they team
up, in order to provide continuity, oversight and guidance for the
young doctor in a setting of fragmented learning. Such a scheme

could provide continuity of observation and care; efficiency; expedited workups; prevention of errors; and perhaps even better than all of those, a less troubled/frightened patient population.

It would help (although this suggestion is impractical for a multitude of reasons) to recognize that learning does not occur at a standard speed for each student. Some individuals learn to be good doctors by spending extra time practicing skill sets repetitively, while others seem quickly to grasp most of the important concepts because they can read faster and retain more than their peers. After all, we accept the idea that surgical techniques are mastered at faster or slower rates depending on manual dexterity as well as the interaction of cerebration and locomotion. Only a rare surgical training program, other than that put in place at Duke by Dr. David Sabiston, has allowed for this self evident truth. The fiscal and personal obstacles to adding time to training, as well as certain other human factors (embarrassment, discouragement, depression, and dishonesty), have been insurmountable.

We must acknowledge that Stead's particular method or style of training, conceived and implemented by one professor-chairman at a single institution, has clearly been dead for several decades, and almost certainly will never be resurrected — at least not in its original construct or intent. I am not aware of the results of the autopsy, if there was one, and I am not certain there has ever been a proper requiem dedicated to the old Stead/Duke way of teaching and learning. More likely than not, we would find that Dr. Stead's system was highly successful in producing uniquely resourceful physicians as well as faculty. In truth, however, there has never been a detailed analysis of results, nor were there any outcome measures in place, so we'll never know for sure.

Those who went through Stead's program love to boast about it and love to recount the treasured trials and tribulations. Being a "Duke Marine" has become something of a cult, in part because today's professors and their training programs across the country are neither unique nor demanding, and most resemble one another closely in terms of hours required, remuneration and extra benefits. Unfortunately, none of them allow individuals to grow their own way. For example, one can't even elect to spend uncounted hours at the bedside or pursue questions by means other than going on line to read at home. I consider the present system to be like an unstable radioisotope; there are lots of emanations, but it would be of interest and great import for all of us to see what the final, stable product looks like—if indeed there ever is one.

At the Heart of Teaching

The results of teaching are definitely unpredictable and certainly unquantifiable. Obviously there is a huge difference between dispersing facts and providing stimulating, unique perspectives. Examples of the latter may be found in that mighty, tiny, paperback book, *Just Say For* Me, containing spoken pronouncements Eugene Stead made during rounds on Osler Ward or in morning report at Duke Hospital. They were collected in the 1960s by two astute house officers, Drs. Fred Schoonmaker (deceased) and Earl Metz, who preserved them in print. Contrast a Stead quotation with usual stuff of teaching rounds: "The art of medicine is not confined to organic disease; it deals with the mind of the patient and with the behavior of a thinking, feeling, human being. The essential skills (of a physician) depend not simply on instruction but on emotional maturity, manifested by sensitive self-cultivation of the ability to see deeply and accurately the problems of another human being...."[1] Compare that to these "rounding pearls": "Her creatinine of 1.1 certifies the presence of renal disease at her age of 70 with loss of most of her muscle mass during long standing weight loss plus wasting." "The serum potassium almost always falls significantly early on when treating diabetic ketoacidosis with an insulin drip; therefore potassium supplements are mandatory." "One measures the QT interval by placing one caliper on the very beginning of the QRS complex and the other caliper at the terminal end of the T wave and not at the terminus of the U wave, when there is one." These last three facts are very important of course, and one will eventually read them during study of a given patient's illness (provided there is time to read!) or hear them during presentation of appropriate patients over the years of rounding. Certainly their delivery during rounds will expedite that particular patient's management and are better remembered when received in the appropriate setting. But if you look closely at portions of Stead's remarks, you can begin to appreciate the value of time in learning: "... essential skills ... depend not simply on instruction ... (but) emotional maturity manifested by ... self-cultivation of ... ability to see ... problems of another human...."

The Value of Extended Time Together

So, how long do you think it could or should take to produce a good doctor? We need to compare the advantages of seeing many patients rather briefly, before they reach Maximal Hospital Benefit (MHB), versus observing far fewer in-patients during a longer course of their illness. In the schema of learning there is something to be said for studying a few patients and their illnesses really well. Surely, today's brief run to MHB wasn't meant in any way to coordinate with either MLB (Maximal Learner's Benefit) or MTB (Maximal Teacher's Benefit). In the design of his training program, Dr. Stead was smart enough to understand that when a young doctor was in the hospital 6 days and 5 nights, he or she was much more likely to be thinking about patients' illnesses, diagnoses and treatments than about a hobby, movie or a game on radio or TV. Obviously if the house officer is called by a nurse about a worrisome change in the patient's course, it is far better for that patient if the nurse is calling a doctor who knows the patient well than if contacting the cross-covering physician. Logistically, it is far easier to go and see a patient that you already know; this continues the learning and more likely than not, provides better care. It certainly bests a course charted by phone without knowing all the facts, especially those garnered by looking at the patient directly. Of course, one can argue that this *modus operandi* doesn't provide much experience in learning how to cross cover, the usual schema for current day practice.

We don't know whether Dr. Stead was smart enough to calculate the number of hours per week required to learn about medicine and about doctoring. Those of us who trained in the Steadian system are often asked: "What did you and your colleagues do with all that time spent in hospital?" The answer is that we had longer intervals at the bedside; more time was allotted to rounding and seeing in detail every patient admitted. Also there were medication reviews on every patient on the ward twice a week, as well as morning rounds with the nurses; all of these caught errors early on. Eating with other physicians in the doctor's dining room or late at night in the cafeteria and isolated from the common distractions of the day made for more doctor talk. Often the Chief Resident made rounds to see the more interesting physical findings from new admissions. Finally, prolonged in-hospital time led to better attendance at the many specialty noon conferences. Not facing a deadline to get home made for an entirely different attitude toward learning.

Any training program worth its salt must expect and demand excellence from every student; must say in one way or another that a young physician's work product is unacceptable when that is the case—because "the professor" expected better and because he knew that the individual was capable of better. You can't say that to a colleague with a straight face unless you have spent many, many hours with a given learner, something that is inconsistently possible in today's rush. A true teacher-learner relationship can never develop in the setting of short hospital stays, too brief attending rotations, and hurried presentations, no longer always at the bedside!

There has not been a construct to adequately replace Stead's Department of Medicine training methods. A specific working solution is unlikely because of democracy in decision-making, and uncertainty about the best possible replacement. Moreover, learners should perhaps have both a voice and a vote in what will be the best training program even while the ACGME exercises several points of control including over the key ingredient or axiom that spending a lot of time with a patient during an episode of illness is necessary for good care and good learning. There is no escaping the fact that the two—care and learning—are obviously linked very tightly. Dr. Stead said, "The rest of the world may be working a four day week, but can you [*really*] be a good doctor [*by practicing*] for four days out of seven only?"[2] (italicized words added to the Stead quotation).

Coda

My remarks here are not the product of scholarly research. They reflect ideas that have originated during decades of reading articles and essays, usually written in anguish and despair, about how best to teach and the obstacles to doing so. Such articles have been published in *JAMA*, the *New England Journal of Medicine*, *Pharos*, and *Journal of General Internal Medicine*. Perhaps the best of these in terms of its title is found in The Lancet: "*Inconvenient Truths About Effective Clinical Teaching.*"[3]

References

1. Stead EA Jr. *Just Say For Me*. Schoonmaker F, Metz E (eds). Denver, CO. World Press, Inc. 1968. p.20.
2. Ibid. p.35.
3. Reilly BM. Inconvenient truths about effective clinical teaching. Lancet. 2007;370(9588):705–11.

Comments Following "Teachers of Medicine and Their Students"

Ruth Ballweg: I agree with Dr. Stead that learning doesn't occur just because there's a teacher in the room teaching. Some teachers might even interfere with learning. I would bet that in any given class, because of different learning styles, probably 20% of the people are infuriated with how the teacher is teaching, and see it as more irritating than helpful. Finally, I'd add that patients are teachers as well.

We haven't really talked much about electronic teaching and electronic learning, and I don't want to suggest that professional schools should move entirely to electronic learning, but some topics lend themselves to that format. There is a whole literature about distance learning with online discussions, especially with students who are decentralized and doing clinical rotations in other places. This creates opportunity for teaching that we are just beginning to explore.

Mort Bogdonoff: I agree with everything that's been said, and I disagree with everything that's been said. It all depends upon the relationship between the teacher and the student. The thing about Gene Stead was that when he beady-eyed you, it had the effect not only of awakening you, but of creating a bond—you knew he was interested. Some teachers might interfere with learning because they're a pain the neck and get in your way.

The notion of using the Internet for teaching leaves out palpability in the business of teaching. At Cornell, pathology is all on the screen. Our students have never actually seen or felt an emphysematous lung, have never held in their hands a heart that's had an infarct. It's a rip-off; it's unbelievable. You've got have palpability.

Bill Stead: I've been known to say that the doctor who can be replaced by a computer, should be. I think my father was saying that the teacher who can be replaced by a computer, should be. I don't think he meant that great teachers were going to be replaced by computers (he didn't think we had many or even any great teachers). The role of the teacher is to inspire and motivate, to get learners excited. My father felt that the teacher needed to provide some sort of a skeleton to help learners navigate, and an active learning environment in which students could explore and pursue problems. One thing that I actually never heard him say but that I think is useful, is that teachers who are great storytellers can, in fact, make extraordinarily complex concepts approachable.

Hal Silberman: Great teachers make the learning fun, memorable, easy, and as permanent as the brain permits. They explain obtuse concepts in a way that even average students understand well enough to explain them to their colleagues. They recognize when a given student needs more time, more teaching and more learning, before moving on in the planned curriculum. And they can criticize in a direct fashion so that the student accepts the criticism, and not only tries harder but improves. To have worked with the student for awhile, there has to be a relationship, as Mort Bogdonoff said.

Elizabeth Ross: A great teacher is someone who loves learning, first of all; someone who loves watching people learn, and teaching students to be lifelong learners. A good teacher promotes internal motivation on the part of the student, rather than external motivation linked to grades or some other force.

Kelly A. Brillant, PA-C, MPH, Clinical Assistant Professor at East Carolina University, met Dr. Stead when he visited ECU's class on "The Role of the PA" every Fall to discuss the importance of midlevel practitioners in healthcare:

The feedback that I get from my students is that great teachers have a passion for what they do, and they demonstrate that passion on rounds and with the students just like Dr. Stead did. This passion is palpable; the students feel it; they know you love your work; they know what you're doing is educating them to become excellent practitioners. I think students follow great teachers into a specialty because they see how rewarding it can be through the eyes of their instructor. Passion: it's magnetic, and students want to feel it as much as their leader does.

Jerome ("Jerry") Ruskin, MD, an intern at Duke in 1960–61, returned from military service in 1963 to complete his residency in medicine and a fellowship in cardiology; he was a faculty member at the time of Dr. Stead's retirement from Duke:

I'm surprised that no one has commented on betting a nickel. One of Dr. Stead's most memorable teaching skills was his ability to inspire you to go and learn on your own, and that was one of his techniques. With a nickel on the line, you really wanted to disprove the professor. Whether you were right or wrong, he wanted you to find the facts, and that has helped me greatly in my practice over the years. I'm sure other people felt the same way. Many things that make a good teacher have already been mentioned, but I had to bring up the nickel. In betting with Dr. Stead, if you lost (the nickel), you still won; if you could trump him, then you won twice.

Doug Zipes: A good teacher is someone you respect, whom you want to emulate. He or she represents the epitome of the profession; whatever they're teaching, you want to be like that person. Dr. Stead was like that.

Michael F. Ball, MD, a Clinical Professor of Medicine at Georgetown, and a Professor of Medicine at Virginia Commonwealth Medical School, INOVA Campus, is now retired from private practice; he was a house officer at Duke with Dr. Stead in the early nineteen-sixties:

One of the things that Dr. Stead instilled in me was the importance of listening to the patient. This is a huge deficit in medical students today. I believe that medical educators must teach students the "art of listening." Dr. Stead used to say to me, "Didn't you listen? Didn't you hear that Mrs. Jones wanted to tell you that?" I did endocrinology before I was a resident. One of our patients had refractory atrial fibrillation, and we talked about all sorts of causes and reasons, and then he just innocently said, "Did you ever ask her if she had a thyroid problem?"

Bill Stead: At one point I went to see my father because I was worried that so many good teachers were leaving Duke. He told me not to worry, saying, "When you're a student and intern, you're really going to like the people who can answer your questions without any hesitation. As you get to be a junior resident and a fellow, you're really going to care about the people that tell you what the real question is." He was saying, "Your judgement about what matters is going to change," and I think that's a very important point. What students want in teachers differs, depending on the phase of their career. They like clarity when they know nothing, and as they begin to know something, they want to understand the questions.

Hal Silberman: How about students who want to become a great doctor in as little time as possible? What does the panel think? Are the students in a rush today, and should they be in a rush to become a great doctor? They have bills to pay, and so forth.

Jeff Wong: Sometimes students come into medical school thinking that way, but it's obviously a pretty naïve and uninformed position. To become a great doctor means a lifetime of work, and some people never achieve it. We agonize a great deal over the medical school curriculum, which lasts four years; we agonize a little bit less over graduate medical education, which lasts anywhere from three to six or seven years; but we don't agonize very much over the 10, 20, 30 years of practice that follow. Continuing medical education is equally, and arguably more, important if people are to keep up and continue to provide good care for patients.

Hal Silberman: I'll take the liberty of suggesting one thing because it happened to me. During my first year of fellowship, my mentor, R. Wayne Rundles, read every single note I dictated on every oncology or hematology patient I saw. The note came back to me with blue marks throughout, and the secretary would have to retype it when revised. It was brutal, but I learned a great deal, certainly about grammar, certainly about thinking and organizing my facts. Students should want that, but I don't know of any teachers who read all those writings.

This is what I think teachers want. They want students to learn well and rapidly, and all at the same rate, while requiring little to no criticism. Now that's the most naïve thing I've said here today. Many people have alluded to the fact that learners don't learn at the same rate, and we make no accommodation for that whatsoever. The curriculum is four years, and at the end of four years, what happens? We've got a doctor, a widget. When I was running the emergency department, certain surgical residents reappeared in the same role that they had occupied a year or two earlier. I asked one who lived nearby me and he said, "Dr. Sabiston, essentially flunked me. He took away one year of my research time and said I had to repeat certain things, and one of them was the rotation in the emergency department." We don't do that in medicine, and I don't think it happens any more in surgery. I don't know how many of you experienced a training program in which one of your peers was asked to repeat a whole rotation.

Doug Zipes: When I was agonizing over a fellowship, I went to Dr. Stead for advice, and he said, "You know, I think you ought to take a fellowship of one week a month for the rest of your life, rather than two years of cardiology."

Hal Silberman: I'm glad you said that. So how long do you think it could, or should take to produce a good doctor?

Andy Wallace: As long as it takes.

Hal Silberman: And yet, we don't do that, do we? Dr. Sabiston did—as long as it takes. It might take six years or longer to become a good resident in surgery. It is likely that some doctors-to-be will require more time than others, and how will we deal with that, given the pathology of the current system. It's too short, but we must make a relationship because in no other way can you discourage the student's bad habits and encourage good ones, and really criticize them in a way that doesn't make him want to go home and shoot himself, or shoot his wife, or kill the dog.

Bill Stead: I think that the way you're saying this brings out the idea that we're going to get the learner to a point, and then stop. There's no good way to do that. The real secret is to somehow change things so that we learn in incremental pieces over our entire career in a way that is as active and effective as we did during my father's tenure when we were in dedicated training. I think figuring out that design gives us the opportunity for the real breakthrough.

Hal Silberman: You don't mean you want me to go to grand rounds and nod off?

Bill Stead: I think grand rounds as they are today can simply be cancelled. That would give us back, what, one hour? Now we've got to figure out what else we can get back. I want us to design the right lifelong learning experience and approach, and I think that will take over. Continuing Medical Education (CME) as we know it is, I believe, totally useless, so I think you've got to think of a completely different model from UME, GME, and CME, using a from-the-ground-up, lifelong, iterative learning.

Donna Shelton, PA-C, who works in out-patient psychiatry in eastern North Carolina, was introduced to Dr. Stead by her father, Bud Shelton, and often traveled with them; Dr. Stead was the one who suggested that she become a PA:

You've just described why I became a PA, because that's how I envisioned my career, my attending always being my mentor, my teacher, and that's what I love about being a PA.

Chuck Hayes: My understanding is that European medical schools, at least at one time, were not so rigidly scheduled, and could last anywhere from four, to six, to eight years. People just did it at their own pace. It seems to me that what students and teachers want more than anything is the opportunity to work in small groups, discussing issues they are assigned to look into and review. At periodic intervals, students and faculty should discuss some of the fine points, because anything you read is somewhat didactic. One needs help with how to think through the issues and discuss them with someone who's done that kind of thinking before. This can become a model for learning how to think. The discussion could concern a specific disease with a lot of information still unknown, or a case presentation, or a complex case discussion like a clinico-pathological conference (CPC). When you do these sorts of things with 100 or 200 people at a time, things get lost in the crowd because there's no opportunity for dialogue. Dialogue facilitates learning, and a lot of what Dr. Stead did was to provide opportunity for dialogue. Unfortunately, since most of us were a little scared of him, we didn't take full advantage of our opportunity.

Patricia Dieter, MPA, PA-C, is Program Director of the Duke University PA Program and Professor, Department of Community and Family Medicine at Duke:

I want to use this opportunity to give you a brief update about what's happened to Dr. Stead's profession. There are now about 150 PA programs nationally, starting from the first one at Duke. And there are international programs, so the concept is spreading throughout the world. Dr. Stead's first PA students, as Dr. Wilson noted, were three ex-Navy corpsmen, and this year we had an entering class of 66, 75% of whom are women, and 25% men. Their average age is 29; they all have bachelor degrees and some have graduate degrees; about 40% have already been licensed or certified in another health profession. It's always fun for me to remind our earlier graduates that our current students are exactly the same age, on average, as the first PA students in the 1960s, and actually have, on average, more patient care experience — about 3½ years, although there's a wide range. They come in with very interesting health care backgrounds, and are a fun group to teach.

I also want to comment about mentoring as a sort of brain-sorting. I think a good teacher is always a mentor. I've been teaching physical diagnosis for 30 years to a variety of students, about 10–12 students each year in a small group. At the end of the course, the students have a final practicum. Immediately after each practicum, I put on my sorting hat, and predict for the student which field of medicine I think they will enter. Since 40 to 50% of Duke PA students come from educationally or economically disadvantaged backgrounds, they have not had the luxury of sorting themselves out or seeing their future in the same way many medical students have; when I predict which field of medicine each student will enter, I think it gives them permission to formulate their own predictions and to dream. A good mentor/teacher recognizes the potential in the learner and starts the sorting process.

Reginald ("Reggie") Carter, PhD, PA, is the former chief of the division of physician assistant education in the Department of Community and Family Medicine at Duke University School of Medicine:

I want to add that North Carolina is one of the top states in the country for PA practice, team delivered practice, and I include nurse practitioners in that, too. Harvey Estes and others have worked hard to make that occur. A good example of how far we have come is that a PA was recently elected as the president of the North Carolina Medical Board. Could anyone have predicted something like that in 1965 when this got started? That's Dr. Stead's legacy, knocking down barriers, keeping our attention centered on the patient, and dealing with problems at hand.

One thing that hasn't been mentioned so far is, above all, to have fun. Dr. Stead had fun working. He told me, "I can't believe they pay me, I have so much fun." He would tell me stories, and you could see the twinkle in his eye. And yes, he could stress you out and could be demanding at times, but if you were around him long enough, you wanted to go back because you had fun. Dr. Stead was a fun-loving person.

Chapter 8

Summing Up the Symposium

Francis A. Neelon, MD, E. Harvey Estes, MD, Andrew G. Wallace, MD

Nearly everyone who passes the crest of life wants to gaze longingly into the retrospectoscope, imaging the days just barely past, seeking to outline the wisdom enveloped in that golden haze. This compulsion appears to have been going on forever; a perhaps apocryphal inscription from a 4800-year old Assyrian tablet states: "The earth is degenerating these days. Bribery and corruption abound. Children no longer mind their parents. Every man wants to write a book and it is evident that the end of the world is fast approaching." Elders always seem to think that the younger generation is losing touch with "their" imperishable values. Those values, being unprovable, take on the texture of self-evident truth to those who have made them into a way of life. The elders feel they profited from exposure to and assimilation of these axioms; they want those who follow to cherish them as well; they bemoan the changes that have come upon their world. But just because the phenomenon is universal does not mean that those lamentations are wrong or misguided. At times the baby *has* been thrown out with the bathwater, at times, the emperor *is* walking naked in the streets. When either happens, a careful review of what has gone on, of what used to be that has been lost or misplaced, can help clarify things and even lead to restoration or reclamation of those values.

This monograph represents the editors' attempt to capture the essence of a day-long symposium held at the Sheraton Imperial

Hotel in Research Triangle Park, North Carolina, on October 26, 2008 in honor of the 100th anniversary of the birth of Eugene A. Stead Jr. The seven invited papers, and an edited version of the comments that followed each of them, are presented in this volume. They illuminate Dr. Stead's profound influence on the teaching of clinical medicine, as well as many of the problems that have beset medical education in the forty years since Dr. Stead relinquished the chair of Medicine at Duke University. Those problems appear to be nearly universally present in American medical schools and teaching hospitals, and no one has articulated any easy solutions. Based on our reading of the Symposium papers and their attending comments, we have tried to distill here the themes running through them, and, following Dr. Stead's advice that we not look back at what is over and done with but rather at what lies ahead of us, we underscore some at least potential solutions for these problems.

Slowing the Hurry of the Hospital

Several contributors to the Symposium note the perceived lack of sufficient time for teaching in American hospitals. House staff (and students) are ejected from the hospital according to a schedule of rigidly enforced duty-hour limitations; harried faculty claim that what time they might have devoted to teaching is consumed by the "need" to earn clinical dollars; professors note that when they do make rounds, the house staff often are absent because they have passed the duty-hour limits and been sent home. Part of our hurry is driven by the desire for large incomes. Earl Metz says in this volume that "the exchange of money for the provision of medical care has changed so much in the past fifty years that it has become the driving force for nearly every aspect of what we do." Is there an answer to this conundrum? Bill Stead points out that his father "and Mother always lived below their income.... My father felt that you should be paid less for thinking because it was enjoyable, and you should be paid more for running in a rat race." It will take a cultural reorientation if we are to recognize that salary dollars exact their price—they tether us to the treadmill of grinding work and obscure "what really counts—taking care of sick people." Perhaps we could start by embracing Gene Stead's crusade to get "the expensive infrastructure [of classroom instruction out] of the medical school, and get it either online or into undergraduate colleges." If medical students started their lives in medicine less burdened by onerous debt, they might look with new eyes on the tasks before them, and be able to resist the blandishments of high-salary-little-time jobs.

Duty hour limitations have been enacted because of legitimate concerns that fatigue impairs the health and safety of tired caregivers and (by implication if not by empirical proof) the health and safety of the patients entrusted to their care. We do need mechanisms that will detect sleepy house staff and students (ideally, that will teach them to recognize and to get sleep when they detect fatigue in themselves), that will provide appropriate places for sleep, and that will insure official encouragement—even insistence—that learners get sufficient sleep. Despite limited hours on duty, it is not certain that forcing house staff to leave the hospital means they will get more sleep or be less error-prone, and this needs further evaluation. But it seems quite clear that duty-hour restriction has had unintended (and deleterious) effects on the curiosity and clinical involvement of learners. Dr. Stead thought that to become proficient in clinical medicine required immersion in the world of the sick, without interruption unless you were pursuing answers (in the library, or in consultation, or in experimentation) to questions that had arisen from interaction with patients. One commonly hears that there are no longer enough young doctors who are willing to commit one or two or three years to such an immersion experience; several of the comments in this volume note an apparent sea-change in attitudes of medical students and young doctors, one that would leave a modern-day Eugene Stead with no learners to teach. We don't think that is the case; we think that if offered the chance, enough will come. We await a brave new professor to put that notion to the test, asking students to sign on for a voyage of wonder and astonishment, but undertaken with a careful eye to their health and welfare while on board.

A willingness to devote the time required to help students master clinical medicine will require a different kind of Professor of Medicine than has recently been in vogue—one who clearly sees and deeply understands the nature of the doctor's job before taking on the teacher's mantle. Being adept in the intricacies of modern biological science is no detriment to such a professor, but alone this will not suffice or even necessarily help; we need department chairs who, like Stead, have lived a real clinical life, not just dabbled in one; who are willing to devote time and energy and their career aspirations to clinical education.

Education, after all, comes to us from the Latin "*ex ducere*" meaning "to draw out." The English synonyms of "education" ("instruct," "school," "drill," "indoctrinate") largely miss this point by looking at what can be put into students rather than what can be led out of them. Socrates recognized the difference when he called himself "a midwife of ideas" and Stead fit this mold; as Chuck Hayes notes in his comments in this volume, Stead, when he became chair of the Department of Medicine, "quit doing research—he went around and checked up on everybody else doing research, but his job was running the teaching program, and he did it magnificently." Stead was willing to make the time to teach; as Andy Wallace notes, "he taught physical diagnosis, he conducted teaching rounds [on Osler Ward] eleven months each year, he took morning report with second year residents and the chief resident, and he regularly attended "Sunday School," the weekly conference where residents … presented what they had learned [from library research]. Gene was deeply interested in the people who trained with him and he spent extended time with them."

Andy Wallace points out in his biographical introduction that Gene Stead was a keen student of how his own mind worked, of how he learned, of how he remembered or forgot. As a result of this introspection, he developed a deep understanding of how people learned—he used that understanding to promote learning in ways that were far ahead of his time, and this guided him in all that he did. Even so, most faculty Stead assembled didn't understand learning at his level, and they suffered from that lack of understanding. One of the bright glimmers today are the few schools that have found ways to preserve selected faculty from the race to make money, and immersed them in faculty development programs that look at how people learn. Those programs and their curricula begin with cognitive neuroscience because they recognize what Stead taught himself: that faculty trained in patient care or research (important and essential as they are) will learn how to motivate learners to learn. We need teachers who have had explicit coaching in how students learn, and environments that emphasize that learning.

Insisting on Responsibility

Duty-hour restrictions mean that a large proportion of house staff and students must be out of the hospital at any given time and, therefore, those left on duty are nominally responsible for the care of too-large numbers of "stranger-patients" (people about whom they are called if problems arise, but whom they have never seen, and may never see—even when they are called about some problem that has arisen in one of the patients they are "cross-covering"). Whether this cross-coverage leads to shoddy care or not remains to be seen, but it surely over-burdens the cross-covering house staff with tasks that cannot be properly accomplished. Because there is too much for any single human to do, there is not time for house officers to even recognize, let alone become, as Andy Wallace says Eugene Stead was, "aware of the complexities of communication between ... doctor and patient." House officers and hospitalist physicians (and the students who look to them for example) have largely become numb or oblivious to what Ruth Ballweg noted was Stead's concern "about the patient's psychosocial history.... about what would happen because the patient was the 'glue' that held her family together." Not on the radar screen of overloaded residents running to stamp our brush fire after brush fire during their nights on call is any hope of glimpsing the importance of the biopsychosocial model in which Bob Klein says Stead operated and which "kept him interested in all the dimensions of the patients on rounds, in all the relationships and psychosocial interactions that set the stage for stress and illness."

Eugene Stead did not want to remove responsibility from young (or old) doctors. Joe Greenfield says in this volume that "indoctrinating the trainee in the essential trait of responsibility was Dr. Stead's primary goal during his teaching rounds.... Dr. Stead's trademark admonition, 'What this patient needs is a doctor,' was most frequently employed because of a trainee's failure to fulfill the role of responsibility toward the patient, not a failure of cognitive function." Bill Stead and several others who commented on Dr. Greenfield's paper note that Dr. Stead instilled responsibility by asking students and resident physicians to know their patients through and through, and to be there to help with the decisions when the patients were sick. To do this, the learners had to be in the hospital and available, had to know the myriad details of their patients' cases, but Stead did not want them "cross-covering" large numbers of patients they did not and would never know. Brit Nicholson points out that "In my experience with Dr. Stead, ... he never left any doubt that that patient in front of me was *my* responsibility; *I* had to be the advocate for that patient." Those entrusted with the education of young doctors must insist that those doctors be personally responsible for the patients in their care, without being loaded down with the treatment of sick people with whom they have no relationship of personal responsibility.

The Widgetification of Medicine

Not directly articulated during the Symposium, but underlying much of the discussion about the pernicious effects of hurry and the problems of too much pseudo-responsibility along with too little of the right kind is the piecework approach to care. Patients are admitted to the hospital because of a narrowly defined medical justification; housestaff and students work feverishly to ameliorate that condition, while ignoring any secondary medical problems the patient may have. This allows the patient to be discharged quickly from the hospital, with the assumption that any loose ends can be tied up by a doctor who has not seen the patient in the hospital, indeed may never have seen him or her before. What is almost certain is that the patient will *not* be seen again by the admitting hospitalist, house officers or students. If the patient articulates a health problem unrelated to the admitting diagnosis, it is consigned to be "worked up as an outpatient" (ie, by somebody else) or turned over to a consultant specialist, who has a similar tunnel vision about what to do and where to do it. Gone are Stead's insistence that each patient was to be examined thoroughly, that the problems unearthed in the process be evaluated, that the charts of every patient be reviewed after discharge for thoroughness and completeness, that every patient cared for primarily by the resident staff be seen, after discharge, in the clinic by the resident who had been responsible for the inpatient episode. Today it seems that each learner sees his or her job in smaller and smaller dimensions, moving furiously to "get this little piece of the work done" as quickly as possible, and move on to the next. Patients feel like they are widgets moving along an assembly line. To be sure, the doctors involved want to be sure that their (self-defined) little part is done very well, that all prescribed treatment conforms to the dictates of "evidence-based medicine," but none of them see the patient whole. As Earl Metz notes, "Dr. Stead carried his own ophthalmoscope and was better at using it than any of us [but] I discovered a couple of years ago that none of our medical residents carries an ophthalmoscope." No student physicians look in eyes, nor in ears; none examine female breasts; it is a rare medical student who has ever seen a rectal or pelvic examination done on the medical floors. Our trainees are moving faster and faster, stamping out widgets, carefully avoiding seeing anything that might lengthen the time before the patient is discharged. It is painfully reminiscent of the "I Love Lucy" episode in the chocolate factory: Lucy and her friend Ethel, working at the chocolate factory, find the assembly line moving faster and faster. In vain attempt to "do their jobs" they resort to stuffing candy in their pockets, their own mouths, their underwear, trying fruitlessly to maintain the semblance of being in control. We need to step back and look carefully at how much our hospitals look like Lucy's candy factory. We need professors who will recognize and figure out how to resist the "tremendous pressure to move patients quickly through the system." We need to heed Harvey Cohen's, and Harvey Estes's, and Chuck Beauchamp's calls to look at teaching arenas other than the hospital. But most of all we need to remember Eugene Stead's insistence that the patient be the center of what we do and the reason why we do it.

Index